A Dictionary of
Medical
and Surgical
Syndromes

A Dictionary of

Medical and Surgical Syndromes

J. Gibson and O. Potparic

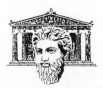

The Parthenon Publishing Group
International Publishers in Medicine, Science & Technology

Casterton Hall, Carnforth,
Lancs, LA6 2LA, UK

120 Mill Road, Park Ridge,
New Jersey 07656, USA

Published in the UK by
The Parthenon Publishing Group Limited
Casterton Hall, Carnforth
Lancs, LA6 2LA, England

Published in the USA by
The Parthenon Publishing Group Inc.
120 Mill Road,
Park Ridge,
New Jersey 07656, USA

British Library Cataloguing-in-Publication Data
Gibson, John
    A dictionary of medical and surgical syndromes.
    I. Title   II. Potparić, Olivera
    610.3

    ISBN 1-85070-338-8

Library of Congress Cataloging-in-Publication Data
Gibson, John. 1907–
        A dictionary of medical and surgical syndromes/J. Gibson and O.
    Potparić.
        p.   cm.
    Includes bibliographical references and index.
    ISBN 1-85070-338-8
    1. Syndromes—Dictionaries.   I. Potparić, O. (Olivera)
    II. Title
    RC69.G53 1991   91-16973
    616' . 047' 03—dc20   CIP

First published 1992

No part of this book may be reproduced
in any form without permission from the publishers except for the quotation of brief
passages for the purposes of review

Phototypesetting by AMA Graphics Ltd., Preston, Lancashire
Printed and bound in Great Britain by
Redwood Press Ltd., Melksham, Wiltshire

Introduction

A syndrome is a group of symptoms and signs or pathological features that form an entity. In essence it is not much different from a disease, and some conditions are referred to sometimes as syndromes sometimes as diseases. In the nineteenth century such a condition was likely to be called a disease; in the twentieth it is likely to be called a syndrome. Some syndromes are called after the doctor or doctors who first described them (Down syndrome, Holmes–Adie syndrome), some after the patient in whom it was first noticed (Hartnup syndrome), some after the clinical or pathological features of the condition (acquired immune deficiency syndrome, carcinoid syndrome), some after a real or fictitious person (Munchausen syndrome, Pickwickian syndrome), some after the place at which it first appeared (Katayama syndrome, Lyme syndrome), some non-committally (X syndrome). Slightly differing versions of some syndromes can appear because the original description may have been altered by later additions or subtraction or other modifications. Many of the congenital syndromes are very rare.

A and V syndrome

These are two types of horizontal strabismus (squint) in which the deviation is significantly different in upward and downward gaze. The terminology is descriptive of the eyes in which deviation is greatest. In A esotropia (deviation of the visual axis of one eye towards that of the other) deviation is greater on eyes up than on eyes down; in A exotropia (deviation of the visual axis of one eye away from the other) deviation is greater on eyes down than on eyes up. In V esotropia, deviation is greater on eyes down than on eyes up; in V exotropia, deviation is greater on eyes up than on eyes down.

Aarskog syndrome

Other name Facio-digital-genital syndrome

Aarskog syndrome is a familial X-linked disorder characterized by short stature, hypertelorism (wide spacing of the eyes), hypoplastic maxilla, short fingers and cryptorchidism (failure of one or both testes to descend into the scrotum). The scrotum often overhangs the penis ('shawl' or 'saddlebag' scrotum).

Aase–Smith syndrome

In Aase–Smith syndrome the thumbs have three phalanges instead of the normal two, and there is hypoplasia of the bone marrow.

Absent abdominal muscle syndrome. See Prune belly syndrome.

Absent pulmonary valve syndrome

Congenital absence of the leaflets of the pulmonary valve can occur in Fallot's tetralogy or be associated with ventricular septal defect or other cardiac congenital lesions. The pulmonary arteries can be grossly dilated and can cause bronchial compression. The arterial duct is usually absent.

Achard syndrome

Achard syndrome is Marfan syndrome with the addition of mandibulo-facial deformities.

Achard–Thiers syndrome

Achard–Thiers syndrome is virilization of women, of adrenocortical origin, associated with hypertension and hyperglycaemia.

Acid aspiration syndrome. See Mendelson syndrome

Acquired immune deficiency syndrome

Other name AIDS

Acquired immune deficiency syndrome is a manifestation of infection with human immunodeficiency virus (HIV), which has affinity for T_4 cells. Once infected a person does not lose the virus. Transmission is by blood, semen, vaginal secretions and, rarely, by breast milk. It is usually transmitted sexually; it is not transmitted by normal social contact. People most likely to be infected are male homosexuals with multiple partners, drug addicts who share needles and syringes, and people who have had a blood transfusion with infected blood. It can be spread by heterosexual intercourse with an infected person. Transmission from mother to child can occur *in utero* and by feeding with infected breast milk.

There is frequently a history of hepatitis in drug addicts who inject drugs intravenously, and in homosexual partners. Homosexual patients may also be infected with gonorrhoea, syphilis and viral enteritis.

Immediately following infection there may be acute influenza-like illness or a glandular fever-like illness. This is followed by a long incubation period of up to 10 years. The full AIDS infection is characterized by a breakdown of immunity, severe opportunistic infections, such as herpes zoster, herpes simplex, perioral or perianal viral infection, *Pneumocystis carinii* pneumonia, and infections of the skin, gastrointestinal tract and central nervous system. Neoplasms such as Kaposi sarcoma, carcinoma of the rectum and squamous cell carcinoma of the mouth can occur. Other features can be fits, depression and a progressive dementia. The disease is fatal, but life can be prolonged by treatment.

Actin dysfunction syndrome

Actin dysfunction syndrome is dysfunction of actin associated with multiple neutrophil abnormalities, recurrent infections and poor responses to inflammation.

Acute nephritic syndrome

Acute nephritic syndrome is characterized by acute microscopic or macroscopic haematuria, proteinuria, oliguria, oedema and impaired renal function. It can follow a postinfectious glomerulonephritis, membrano-proliferative glomerulonephritis or immunoglobulin gamma A nephropathy after an interval of 20–60 days. It can occur at any age, but is most common in children and adolescents and it can occur in small epidemics. It can also occur as a complication of polyarteritis nodosa, systemic lupus erythematosus and Wegener granulomatosis. Most patients recover within 2–3 weeks, but proteinuria can persist for several years. Complications are nephrotic syndrome, pulmonary oedema, encephalopathy and a deterioration in renal function.

Acute radiation syndrome

Acute radiation syndrome follows exposure to a large amount of radiation. Vomiting begins in about 12 hours and is followed by fever, diarrhoea, prostration, purpura and petechial spots. About 5 days later collapse, tachycardia, hypotension and bloody diarrhoea occur. Death is likely in 7–10 days after exposure.

Acute relapsing Landry–Guillain–Barré syndrome

Recurrence of the Landry–Guillain–Barré syndrome can occur after an asymptomatic interval of months or years and is characterized by a progressive weakness lasting for 1–3 weeks, followed by recovery.

Adams–Oliver syndrome

Adams–Oliver syndrome is a variable autosomal dominant condition in which there is aplasia of the scalp and skull bones with reduction in length of the distal limbs.

Adams–Stokes syndrome. See Stokes–Adams syndrome

Addison–Schilder syndrome

Other name Adrenoleukodystrophy

Addison-Schilder syndrome is due to cerebral demyelination occurring in the first two decades of life in a patient with Addison disease. It is probably a sex-linked recessive disorder. The neurological consequences can be blindness, deafness, hemiplegia, quadriplegia, pseudobulbar palsy and dementia.

Adie syndrome. See Holmes–Adie syndrome

Adrenogenital syndrome. See Congenital adrenogenital syndrome

Adult respiratory distress syndrome

Other names Shock lung; post-traumatic pulmonary insufficiency; congestive atelectasis

Respiratory distress syndrome can arise in the post-shock period. It is characterized by a gradually increasing intrapulmonary venous admixture during the first few days after the insult. Hypoxia in the presence of normal filling pressures and a clear X-ray of the chest may be the first evidence of septic shock. With progression, bilateral diffuse pulmonary infiltrates appear on the chest X-ray. There is an inability to maintain adequate arterial oxygenation in spite of high inspired concentrations of oxygen. Though the aetiology of the condition is uncertain, many factors are probably involved, including decreased perfusion of the lung (with micro-infarcts), trauma to the chest, oxygen toxicity and fat embolism. It can appear as a complication of *Plasmodium falciparum* infection.

AEC syndrome

AEC syndrome is an autosomal dominant condition characterized by:

  A – ankyloblepharon (adhesion of the ciliary edges of the eyelids to each other)
  E – ectodermal defects
  C – cleft lip (palate).

Associated features can be absent or dystrophic nails, sparse wire-like hair or alopecia, pointed widely-spaced teeth, a broad bridge to the nose, a recessed maxilla and decreased sweating.

Afebrile pneumonitis syndrome

Afebrile pneumonitis syndrome is a perinatally acquired pneumonia occurring in infants under 4 months of age. It is thought to be due to colonization of the infant's nasopharynx or conjunctiva with micro-organisms acquired from the mother's vagina during birth. The organisms can be *Pneumocystis carinii, Chlamydia trachomatis, Ureaplasma urealyticum, Mycoplasma hominis* and cytomegalovirus; often more than one of them is involved. Clinical features are an afebrile infection with rapid breathing, cough and congestion. Severe respiratory distress can occur. X-ray of the lungs shows bilateral hyperaeration, frequently with atelectasis and infiltration. The infection responds to treatment, but the infant may be left with some degree of pulmonary dysfunction.

Afferent loop syndrome

Afferent loop syndrome is duodenal distension, abdominal pain and nausea due to chronic partial obstruction of the duodenum following gastrojejunostomy.

Afzelius syndrome. See Immotile cilia syndrome

Albatross syndrome

Albatross syndrome refers to a patient 'hanging about the surgeon's neck' (from Coleridge, S.T. *The Rime of the Ancient Mariner*) with numerous complaints following a failure of gastric surgery in a wrongly selected patient.

Albright syndrome

Other names Polyostotic fibrous dysplasia; McCune–Albright syndrome

Albright syndrome (which does not seem to be heritable, but has been reported in monozygotic twins) is characterized by osteitis fibrosa disseminata (a fibrous dysplasia of several bones which can induce pathological fractures) and melanotic macules in the skin present at birth or appearing in neonatal life, usually unilateral and seen especially on the forehead, the back of the neck, the sacral region and the buttocks. Other features can be endocrine dysfunction and precocious puberty. Frequency is about the same in both sexes.

Alcohol withdrawal syndrome

Sudden withdrawal of alcohol can cause tremor, fits, hallucinations, a confusional state, nausea, vomiting, tachycardia, vasodilatation and anorexia. When all or most of these features are present the condition is called delirium tremens.

Aldrich syndrome. See Wiskott–Aldrich syndrome

Alexia without agraphia syndrome

Alexia without agraphia syndrome is one of the 'disconnection syndromes' of the brain. A lesion of the left occipital lobe and the splenium of the corpus callosum prevents information that has been fed into the right occipital lobe from reaching the left hemisphere. The results are that the patient has alexia (inability to read), an inability to name colours and an inability to copy writing, but is able to write spontaneously and to identify colours.

Alezzandrini syndrome

Alezzandrini syndrome is characterized by loss of hair pigment from the eyebrows and eyelashes, facial vitiligo (patches of depigmentation), deafness and unilateral retinal degeneration.

Algid malaria syndrome

Algid malaria syndrome is an acute shock syndrome occurring in malaria due to *Plasmodium falciparum*. There is a vascular collapse. The blood pressure may be so low that it cannot be measured; the pulse is rapid and may be so feeble that it cannot be felt. These symptoms can occur at the beginning of the infection or during treatment or they may indicate the onset of a gram-negative septicaemia.

Alpha chain syndrome

Alpha chain syndrome is a disease of the Arabian peninsula and the Eastern Mediterranean, characterized by a severe enteropathy and finger clubbing. The intestinal mucosa is infiltrated with plasma producing only heavy chain immunoglobulin A (IgA).

Alport syndrome

Other name Hereditary nephritis with deafness

Alport syndrome is a familial disorder characterized by sensorineural deafness, nephritis and eye abnormalities. It is thought to be due to an autosomal inherited defect of the glomerular basement membrane of the kidneys. The renal disease is apparent at an early age, and recurrent haematuria is common. Eye abnormalities include spherophakia (spherical lens), lenticonus (congenital bulging forwards of the lens), cataracts and glaucoma. Males are more frequently affected than are females. It may account for up to 3% of cases of chronic renal failure in children.

Variants of the disease are associated with diabetes mellitus, icthyosis, polyneuropathy, myopathy and Bernard–Soulier (giant platelet) syndrome.

Alström syndrome

Alström syndrome is an inherited disease involving the ear, eye, kidney and endocrine glands. An affected child is obese, has nerve deafness and retinal degeneration ('atypical retinitis pigmentosa') and becomes blind by the age of 7 years. In an adult, carbohydrate intolerance is slowly progressive, the obesity may disappear and renal disease can develop and progress to renal failure. A male patient will show an unusual primary hypogonadism with small testes, low plasma testosterone, elevated gonadotrophin levels but normal secondary sexual characteristics. A female patient may show no evidence of hypogonadism, but menstruation may be irregular. Other features can be baldness, scoliosis, hyperostosis frontalis, acanthosis nigricans, hyperuricaemia and hypertriglyceridaemia.

Amniotic band syndrome

Amniotic band syndrome is due to the formation of amniotic bands between the fetus and a sticky chorion due to the loss of some amnion early in pregnancy. There is an increased risk in Ehlers–Danlos syndrome and Marfan syndrome. By constricting the limbs these bands can cause oedema beyond the constriction, terminal syndactyly and limb amputations.

Anderson–Fabry syndrome. See Fabry syndrome

Anterior chest wall syndrome

Anterior chest wall syndrome is a sharp localized tenderness of intercostal muscles. It can be associated with functional disorders such as anxiety, palpitations, hyperventilation, headache and feelings of exhaustion. It can be mistaken for angina pectoris, but angina pectoris due to coronary insufficiency is not associated with tenderness of the chest wall.

Anterior cord syndrome

A lesion of the anterior parts of the spinal cord produces motor weakness and loss of pain sense and temperature sense below the level of the lesion.

Anterior spinal artery syndrome

Other name Beck syndrome

Occlusion of the anterior spinal artery causes quadriplegia if the occlusion is at the upper end of the spinal cord, or a flaccid paralysis of the legs with dissociated sensory loss if it is at the lower end. The syndrome may follow periods of hypotension, especially in elderly patients. It can also be due to infarction of the anterior spinal artery following ossification of the posterior longitudinal ligament of the spinal column.

Anterior tibial syndrome

Other names Tibialis anterior syndrome; March syndrome

Raised pressure and pain in the anterior Tibial compartment followed by necrosis of muscle, due to excessive walking or marching.

See also Compartmental syndrome

Antihypertensive drug withdrawal syndrome

Other names Antihypertensive drug discontinuation/rebound syndrome

Antihypertensive drug withdrawal syndrome is due to a sudden cessation of therapy of antihypertensive drugs of the centrally-acting type such as clonidine, guanfacine and α-methyldopa. The syndrome is characterized by symptoms of sympathetic overactivity, increased heart rate, raised blood pressure, tremor, anxiety and insomnia. Symptoms appear 18–21 hours after the cessation of treatment, and they last for 1–5 days. The severity and incidence are dose-dependent. It is prevented by not stopping treatment abruptly.

Anton syndrome

The denial of blindness by a cortically blind patient with a lesion of the occipital lobes.

Anxiety syndrome

Anxiety syndrome is characterized by nervousness, trembling, sweating, rapid pulse, rapid and shallow breathing, dry mouth and palpitations, produced by severe anxiety.

Antiphospholipid antibody syndrome

Antiphospholipid antibodies (lupus anticoagulant antibody and anti-cardiolipin antibody) can produce a syndrome with a partial overlap with systemic lupus erythematosus. They are associated with arterial occlusion (especially of the ocular and ophthalmic arteries), venous thromboses and thrombocytopenia and, less commonly, with valvular disease of the heart, migraine, chorea and livedo reticularis. They are a serious risk in pregnancy: in a pregnant woman there is an increased liability of arterial occlusion, venous thrombosis, thrombocytopenia, fetal growth retardation, intrauterine death, abortion or premature delivery.

Aortic arch syndrome

Other names Takayasu syndrome; Takayasu aortitis; pulseless disease; brachial arteritis; brachocephalic aortitis

Aortic arch syndrome is a non-specific inflammatory disease of arteries affecting mainly the aorta and its main branches and causing obstruction of the blood flow. The carotid pulses and the pulses in the arm may be absent.

Apert syndrome

Other name Acrocephalosyndactyly

Apert syndrome is a congenital disorder characterized by oxycephaly (a congenital deformity of the skull, which rises to a peak), associated with syndactylism and mental retardation. Other features can be hypertelorism, strabismus, proptosis, downward slanting of the palpebral fissures, low-set ears, submucous cleft palate, malocclusion of teeth and a ventricular septal defect.

Arnold–Chiari syndrome

Other name Chiari–Arnold syndrome

Arnold–Chiari syndrome is a herniation of the medulla oblongata and sometimes part of the cerebellum through the foramen magnum. It is commonly associated with a meningocele or a meningomyecele and can cause hydrocephalus.

Asherman syndrome

Synechiae developing within the uterus after curettage can cause amenorrhoea and infertility.

Asperger syndrome

Other name Autistic psychopathy

Asperger syndrome is a serious disorder of childhood resembling autism and thought by some to be a subgroup of that condition and not a clinical entity. Clinical features include abnormal speech (which can be lengthy, pedantic and stereotyped), impaired non-verbal communication, lack of empathy, repetitive activities, resistance to change, clumsy or stereotyped movements and areas of intensive preoccupation in specialized subjects such as dinosaurs, computers, electronics and outer space.

See also Kanner syndrome

Asplenia syndrome

Other name Ivemark syndrome

Asplenia syndrome is a congenital syndrome characterized by absence of the spleen, transposition of the viscera, transposition of the great arteries, and congenital heart defects. The aetiology is unknown. Death occurs at an early age.

Ataxia–telangiectasia syndrome

Ataxia–telangiectasia syndrome is an autosomal recessive disorder with an incidence of 2 to 3 per 100 000 live births. Clinical features are ataxia, telangiectasia (enlarged clumps of blood vessels), chronic sinus and pulmonary disease, variable B-cell and T-cell deficiency, and endocrine abnormalities.

The ataxia is progressive and is due to a progressive degeneration of neurons of the cerebellar cortex. It is usually the presenting feature and becomes apparent when the child starts to walk. Other neurological features are progressive muscular weakness, choreo-athetosis, intention tremor, nystagmus, dysarthria and a failure of intellectual development over the age of 9 years. The telangiectasia appear in the conjunctiva, nose, ears and shoulders. Other skin anomalies are atrophy of the skin, premature greying of the hair, vitiligo or *café au lait* spots, multiple keratoses and basal cell carcinoma. T-cell deficiency causes lymphopenia; B-cell deficiency causes absence of IgA and IgE. Endocrinological defects are hypoplasia of the ovaries, cytoplasmic vacuoles in the anterior pituitary and elevated gonadotrophin. Recurrent infections are common. The prognosis is poor, with death usually due to pneumonia or bronchiectasis.

Autoerythrocyte sensitization syndrome

See Gardner–Diamond syndrome

Avellis syndrome

Avellis syndrome is paralysis of the soft palate and vocal cords on one side and loss of pain sensation and temperature sense on the other side due to a lesion of the nucleus ambiguus and spinothalamic tract.

Awake apnoea syndrome

Awake apnoea syndrome is a non-epileptic seizure occurring in infants who may have a history of regurgitation: a lower oesophageal pH study may show evidence of a gastro-oesophageal reflux. It occurs in an awake infant who has been fed within an hour and then placed in a supine or sitting position. Suddenly the infant stops breathing for a few moments, stares, goes into a rigid opisthotonic posture (the head and heels being bent backwards and the body bowed forward) and then develops hypotonia and cyanosis or pallor. The child does not choke, cough or gag. The cyanosis or pallor can last for up to 30 minutes.

Axenfeld syndrome

Axenfeld syndrome is characterized by glaucoma, hypertelorism (wide spacing of the eyes), hypoplasia of the malar bones, congenital absence of some teeth and mental retardation.

Ayerza syndrome

Ayerza syndrome is characterized by cyanosis, polycythaemia, and heart failure, due to chronic pulmonary insufficiency and sclerosis of the pulmonary vascular bed.

B

Balint syndrome

Balint syndrome is a disorder of oculomotor function due to bilateral lesions of the parietal and occipital lobes. Clinical features include spasm of fixation, optic ataxia (an inability to touch or grasp an object offered) and simultanagnosia (perception of parts of a picture or pattern but inability to recognize the whole).

Balint–Holmes syndrome

Balint–Holmes syndrome is visual disorientation due to bilateral lesions of the parietal lobes.

Baller–Gerold syndrome

Baller–Gerold syndrome is a familial recessive disorder characterized by craniosynostosis and hypoplasia or absence of a radius.

Bannwarth syndrome

Bannwarth syndrome is a lymphocytic meningoradiculitis due to infection by *Borrelia burgdorferi*, the cause of Lyme syndrome.

Banti syndrome

Banti syndrome is characterized by portal hypertension with congestive splenomegaly, with which can be associated anaemia, leukopenia, cirrhosis of the liver, gastrointestinal haemorrhage, oedema, ascites, muscle wasting, spider naevi and liver palms. Mental impairment and a flapping tremor of the hands are a result of hepatic encephalopathy.

Barlow syndrome. See Prolapsed mitral valve syndrome

Barr–Shaver–Carr syndrome. See XXXY syndrome

Bartter syndrome

Bartter syndrome is due to juxtaglomerular and renomedullary cell hyperplasia. Clinical features present in infancy or childhood and include anorexia, failure to thrive, polydipsia, polyuria and muscle weakness. Other features can be rickets, tetany, fits, hypercalcaemia, hypophosphataemia, distal renal tubular acidosis, renal failure, growth retardation and mental retardation.

Basal cell naevus syndrome. See Gorlin syndrome

Basan syndrome

Basan syndrome is an autosomal dominant condition characterized by coarse scalp hair, which is shed during the second decade of life, sparse eyebrow lashes and body hair, severe dental caries, decreased sweating and dry skin and mucous membranes.

Basex syndrome

Other name Paraneoplastic acrokeratosis

Psoriasiform plaques develop on the face, hands and feet, the palmar and plantar skin is thickened and the nails become dystrophic and break easily. It is associated with carcinoma of the pharynx or larynx.

Bassen–Kornzweig syndrome

Other name Abetalipoproteinaemia

Bassen–Kornzweig syndrome is an autosomal recessive inherited condition in which there is a reduction or absence of β-lipoproteins. Affected infants have diarrhoea, steatorrhoea, malabsorption and areflexia. Later clinical features are spinocerebellar degeneration, ptosis, strabismus, peripheral neuropathy, ataxia, retinal degeneration, cardiac arrhythmias and failure and acanthocytosis (abnormally-shaped red cells with a thorny appearance).

Battered baby syndrome

Other names Non-accidental injury; Caffey syndrome

Battered baby syndrome is a syndrome of repeated injuries inflicted on a baby or young child by a parent or other adult. Injuries can be bruises, cigarette burns, burns from electric fires, scalds, eye haemorrhages, fractures, subdural haematomas, brain damage, ruptured liver, ruptured spleen and torn mesentery. Malnutrition and other signs of child neglect and cruelty can be present.

Bazzana syndrome

Bazzana syndrome is characterized by deafness due to a progressive otosclerosis associated with visual impairment due to contracture of the visual fields.

Beck syndrome. See Anterior spinal artery syndrome

Beckwith–Wiedemann syndrome

Other names Beckwith syndrome; visceromegaly syndrome

Beckwith–Wiedemann syndrome is an autosomal condition characterized by high birth weight, omphalocele (hernia into the umbilical cord), macroglossia, enlarged liver and spleen, hyperplasia of the kidney, congenital abnormalities of the urinary tract, slight microcephaly, and a susceptibility to develop benign and malignant tumours, especially rhabdomyosarcoma and Wilm tumour. Pancreatic island cell hyperplasia can cause hyperinsulinaemia and hypoglycaemia. The infant may show an excessive insulin response to intravenous glucose, which results in further hypoglycaemia. The liability to develop hypoglycaemia is usually lost as the infant grows older.

Behçet syndrome

Behçet syndrome is a disease of unknown origin, possibly HLA-B5 associated, most common in the Eastern Mediterranean countries and in Japan. It is a chronic relapsing disease, involving many systems, and can be fatal. Common clinical features are iritis (which can progress to blindness) and apthous ulcers of the mouth and genitalia. Other features can be thrombophlebitis, fever, gastrointestinal ulceration, arthropathy, myelitis, aseptic meningitis, a syndrome resembling benign intracranial hypertension, convulsions, stupor, an encephalitis-like illness with delirium, and a stroke due to a sudden neurological involvement. The skin can show hypergy (the liability of sterile blisters to develop at venepuncture sites).

Behr syndrome

Behr syndrome consists of familial spastic paraplegia with or without optic atrophy.

21

Benedict syndrome

Other name Benedikt syndrome

Infarction or a tumour involving the red nucleus, the third cranial nerve and the corticospinal tract causes oculomotor paralysis and ataxia on the same side and tremor and paralysis of the arm and leg on the opposite side.

Bernard–Soulier syndrome

Other name Giant platelet syndrome

Bernard–Soulier syndrome is an abnormality of blood platelets in which there is an absence or deficiency of platelet glycoprotein-1 from the platelet membrane. The platelets are much enlarged, reduced in number and defective in binding coagulation factors. Bleeding episodes can occur.

Bertolotti syndrome

Bertolotti syndrome is an association of sciatic pain with sacralization of the fifth lumbar vertebra (fusion of the vertebra with the sacrum).

Bickers–Adams syndrome

Bickers–Adams syndrome is an X-linked stenosis of the cerebral aqueduct which causes hydrocephalus.

BIDS syndrome

BIDS syndrome is an autosomal recessive inherited disease characterized by:

    B – brittle hair
    I – impairment, physical and mental
    D – decreased fertility
    S – short stature

See also IBIDS syndrome

Biglieri syndrome

In Biglieri syndrome deficiency of cortisol, androgen and oestrogens is due to deficiency of 17-hydroxylase.

Biörck syndrome

In Biörck syndrome an argentaffinoma (a carcinoid tumour of the gastrointestinal tract) is associated with pulmonary stenosis and cyanotic flushing.

Bjornstad syndrome

Bjornstad syndrome is an autosomal dominant inherited condition of pili torti (twisted hairs) which is associated with nerve deafness.

B–K mole syndrome. See Familial atypical multiple mole-melanoma syndrome

Blackfan–Diamond syndrome. See Josephs–Diamond–Blackfan syndrome

Black locks, albinism, deafness syndrome

Other name BADS

The hair and skin are white as a result of an absence of melanin, except for some black locks of hair and some brown macules in the skin. There is a congenital neurosensorial deafness.

Bland–Garland–White syndrome

Left ventricular failure occurring shortly after birth is due to the left coronary artery arising from the pulmonary artery and not from the aorta. If untreated, death is likely in childhood or adolescence.

Blegvadt–Haxthausen syndrome

In Blegvadt–Haxthausen syndrome osteogenesis imperfecta (brittle bone syndrome) is associated with anetoderma (abnormal looseness and atrophy of the skin).

Blind loop syndrome

Other name Stagnant loop syndrome

The characteristic features of Blind loop syndrome are abdominal pain, diarrhoea, steatorrhoea (excess of faecal fat), vitamin B_{12} deficiency, and loss of weight. As a result of an operation on the small intestine, a segment of it has a blind end in which the contents are stagnant, or stagnation can be due to a stricture. Steatorrhoea is mainly due to an interference with bile salt metabolism. Bacterial action on tryptophan causes the production of excessive amounts of indican and indole. The contents of the blind loop become infected with micro-organisms such as bacteroides, which utilize vitamin B_{12} and so cause vitamin B_{12} deficiency.

The syndrome can also occur in patients with a jejunal diverticulum, a gastrocolic fistula, a gastrojejunocolic fistula or a duodenocolic fistula.

Bloch–Sulzberger syndrome

Other name Incontinentia pigmenti

Bloch–Sulzberger syndrome is an autosomal recessive disorder, occurring mainly in females. A vesiculobullous eruption is present at birth or develops within 2 weeks; development can occur later in life. From the 12th week of life hyperpigmentation of the skin develops, especially in the lateral regions of the trunk and in the perimammary areas. After the age of 2 years the pigmentation starts to fade. Other features can be cataracts, strabismus, optic nerve atrophy, blue sclerae, scarring alopecia, spoon-shaped nails, short stature, spina bifida, cleft lip and palate, microcephaly, spastic paralysis, hydrocephalus, teeth and ear abnormalities, cardiac abnormalities and mental retardation. Over 15% of patients become blind.

Bloom syndrome

Bloom syndrome is an autosomal recessive inherited condition most common in Ashkenazi Jews. There is a defect in DNA replication. It is characterized by low birth weight, short stature, dolicoephalic (long) skull, a characteristic face with a narrow prominent nose, a receding chin and hypoplastic malar region, telangiectatic erythema of the face and photosensitivity. *Café au lait* spots are present in about half the patients. Multiple severe infections of the gastrointestinal tract and respiratory tract are common. There is an increased incidence of leukaemia, lymphoma, lymphosarcoma and carcinoma of the mouth and gastrointestinal tract. Sexual development is normal but males are infertile owing to sperm defects. The intelligence is usually normal and neurological abnormalities are uncommon. Immunoglobulin levels are low and chromosomal abnormalities of various kinds are present.

Blue diaper syndrome

A defect of tryptophan transport across the small intestine wall causes tryptophan to be degraded by bacteria to indoles which are absorbed. The diapers of affected infants can become blue due to an interaction between bleach and urinary indican. Later features are mental retardation, hypercalcaemia and nephrocalcinosis.

Blue rubber bleb naevus syndrome

Blue rubber bleb naevus syndrome is an autosomal dominant inherited condition in which there are blue cavernous haemangioma in the skin. They are about 3–4 centimetres in diameter and feel like rubber. They can be painful. Excessive sweating can occur. Similar haemangioma are present in the gastrointestinal tract and can, by bleeding, cause melaena.

Bobble-head doll syndrome

Bobble-head doll syndrome is continuous bobbing up and down of the head of a child with hydrocephalus or a large third ventricle cyst.

'Body-all-aching-and-racked-with-pain' syndrome

Severe muscular pain and aching all over the body can follow anaesthesia by suxamethonium. The pain is of uncertain origin but may be due to muscular fasciculation. It is most likely to occur in women, middle-aged patients and unfit patients. It can occur immediately after the anaesthetic or not until the 3rd or 4th postanaesthetic day. It usually lasts for 3–4 days.

Boerhaave syndrome

Boerhaave syndrome is a spontaneous rupture of the oesophagus, usually occurring during vomiting, and associated with incoordinated oesophageal contractions.

Bonnet–Dechaume syndrome

In Bonnet–Dechaume syndrome a vascular malformation of the brainstem is conjoined to a cirsoid aneurysm of the retina.

Böök syndrome

Other name PHC syndrome

Böök syndrome is an autosomal dominant inherited condition character- ized by absence or partial absence of the tricuspid teeth, premature whitening of the hair of the scalp, axillae and pubic region, and excessive sweating of the palms and soles.

Borjeson–Forssman–Lehman syndrome

Borjeson–Forssman–Lehman syndrome is an X-linked recessive syndrome characterized by obesity, hypopituitarism, hypogonadism, narrow palpebral fissures, epilepsy and mental retardation.

Bourneville syndrome

Other names Tuberous sclerosis; epiloia

Bourneville syndrome is characterized by severe mental retardation associated with adenoma sebaceum (overgrowth of the sebaceous glands) of the face, tuberous sclerosis of the brain, tumours of the heart and kidney, and epilepsy.

Bradycardia–tachycardia syndrome. See Sick sinus syndrome

Brain damage behaviour syndrome

Lesions of the brain in those areas concerned with behaviour and language function can cause disinhibition, hyperactivity, catastrophic reactions and deficiency in language concepts and number concepts. The speech defect is commonly one of a disturbance of the language–symbol association. Expressive aphasia is common. An affected child can understand language but cannot reproduce it. Receptive aphasia can be severe; the child cannot interpret language symbols. A combination of expressive and receptive aphasia is called mixed aphasia.

Brainstem syndromes

In brainstem syndromes cranial nerve palsies are associated with motor and sensory disturbance on the other side of the body (as the motor and sensory pathways cross at a lower level), and they are usually due to an infarction of the brainstem or a tumour involving it.

Briquet syndrome

Briquet syndrome is a disorder beginning before the age of 30 years and is more common in women than in men. The patient reports multiple physical complaints for which there is no physical evidence and which cause her or him to lead a life of semi-invalidism, with many calls upon a doctor.

Brittle bone syndrome

Other name Osteogenesis imperfecta

Brittle bone syndrome is a genetic disease of collagen characterized by brittle bones, frequent fractures, short stature, macrocephaly, thin skin and blue sclerae. Otosclerotic deafness can occur.

See also van der Hoeve syndrome

Broad thumb syndrome. See Rubinstein–Taybi syndrome

Brock syndrome

Other name Middle lobe syndrome

Brock syndrome is collapse and pneumonitis of the middle lobe of the right lung due to compression of the middle lobe bronchus by enlarged lymph nodes, usually tuberculous.

Bronze baby syndrome

Bronze baby syndrome is due to phototherapy of infants and may be induced by the photoxidation products of bilirubin. The skin develops a grey–brown discoloration, direct hyperbilirubinaemia develops and the serum and urine have a dirty-grey colour.

Brown bowel syndrome

Other name Intestinal ceroidosis

In Brown bowel syndrome a brown pigment (ceroid or lipofuscin) is deposited in the smooth muscle cells of the alimentary tract. It is associated with vitamin E deficiency, which can occur in malnutrition, cirrhosis of the liver, cystic fibrosis, biliary atresia, chronic pancreatitis and hypoproteinaemia. An intestinal pseudo-obstruction can occur.

Brown-Séquard syndrome

Hemisection of the spinal cord can cause: (a) paralysis and sensory loss in the muscles and skin supplied from the affected segment; (b) spastic paralysis and loss of vibration sense and position sense on the same side; (c) loss of pain sense and temperature sense on the other side. Complete hemisection is rare. A partial syndrome can occur in multiple sclerosis.

Bruns syndrome

Paroxysmal headache, vomiting and giddiness on movement of the head and sometimes falling can be caused by a cyst of the fourth cerebral ventricle or other lesions causing obstruction to the flow of cerebrospinal fluid.

Brusa–Torricelli syndrome

In Brusa–Torricelli syndrome aniridia (congenital absence of the iris) and other congenital defects are associated with a neuroblastoma.

Budd–Chiari syndrome

Other name Chiari syndrome

Budd–Chiari syndrome is characterized by cirrhosis of the liver and ascites due to an obstruction of the hepatic vein by a blood clot or tumour. The portal and splenic veins increase in diameter and are more undulating than usual. The spleen and liver are nearly always enlarged, and jaundice and ascites can occur.

Burnett syndrome. See Milk-alkali syndrome

Buschke–Ollendorff syndrome

In this autosomal dominant inherited condition there is an abnormality of elastin. Clinical features are osteopoikilosis (a mottled appearance of bone due to multiple sclerotic foci) and yellowish papules in the skin.

Butler–Albright syndrome

Other, name Adult-type distal renal tubular acidosis

Butler–Albright syndrome is a sporadic or autosomal dominant inherited form of renal tubular acidosis. The onset is usually over the age of 2 years. Early clinical features are vomiting, anorexia, constipation and dehydration. Later features are nephrocalcinosis, interstitial nephritis, renal stones and renal failure. Osteomalacia can develop and cause pathological fractures. Potassium loss and hypokalaemia can cause weakness and periodic paralyses. Other features can be respiratory difficulties, cardiac arrhythmias, flaccid paralysis and growth retardation. With early diagnosis and treatment the prognosis can be good if the more severe complications can be prevented.

Bywaters syndrome. See Crush syndrome

C

Caffeine withdrawal syndrome

Headache can be due to giving up drinking coffee or following a switch from ordinary coffee to decaffeinated coffee. Muscle pain and tiredness can also occur.

Caffey syndrome. See Battered baby syndrome

Caffey–Silverman syndrome

Other name Infantile cortical hyperostosis

Caffey–Silverman syndrome is a familial disease of infants characterized by hyperostoses, swelling of tissues over affected bones, irritability and fever.

Calf pump failure syndrome

Other names Postphlebetic syndrome; postphlebetic leg; postthrombotic leg

Calf pump syndrome is characterized by oedema of the legs (absent on getting up, getting worse as the day progresses), degenerative changes and irritation and pain in the skin of the leg, recurrent and often painful ulceration above the medial malleolus, and venous claudication (a bursting pain in the calf after walking for some time) and sometimes a 'champagne-bottle' leg due to constriction of the tissues by a band of liposclerosis just above the ankle. Varicose veins may be present.

It is usually due to a deep-vein thrombosis of veins beneath the deep fascia of the leg; it can be due to paralysis or atrophy of the calf muscles after a stroke. It is a failure of the calf muscle pump, which normally aids the return of venous blood from the leg by its contractions. It can occur shortly after the thrombosis or not for several years.

Camurati–Engelmann syndrome

Camurati–Engelmann syndrome is a familial dominant condition characterized by fusiform enlargement of the shafts of the bone of the legs, other bony deformities, eye defects and hypogonadism.

Canada–Cronkhite syndrome

Other name Cronkhite–Canada syndrome

Canada–Cronkhite syndrome is characterized by multiple gastrointestinal polyps, hypermelanosis of the skin (and in some patients of the lips and mucous membrane of the mouth), abdominal pain, diarrhoea, malnutrition, hair loss and nail atrophy.

Canavan syndrome

Canavan syndrome is an autosomal recessive inherited disease in which a spongy degeneration of the white matter of the brain develops in infancy and causes optic atrophy with blindness, muscle rigidity, poor head control and exaggerated reflexes. The head can become enlarged. Death usually occurs in the first 5 years of life.

Candidiasis–endocrinopathy syndrome

Candidiasis–endocrinopathy syndrome is an autoimmune disorder in which organ-specific antibodies against a variety of endocrine glands can appear early. Clinical features are a mucocutaneous monilial infection, which is evident soon after birth, hypoparathyroidism and adrenal insufficiency. Sprue and pernicious anaemia are complications.

Caplan syndrome

In Caplan syndrome rheumatoid arthritis is associated with a nodular fibrosis of the lungs in miners.

Capgrass syndrome

Other name Illusion of doubles

The patient is deluded that a person, usually a close relative, has been replaced by an exact double. There can be ambivalent feelings towards the 'double'. It is a feature of paranoid schizophrenia, can be associated with de Clérambault syndrome, and can occur as an early feature of dementia in elderly patients. An organic basis is likely.

As a variant of this syndrome the patient believes that inanimate objects, such as furniture, a letter, a watch, spectacles, have been replaced by an exact double.

Carcinoid syndrome

Carcinoid syndrome is produced by an excessive secretion of serotonin (5-hydroxytryptamine) by a carcinoid tumour of the appendix (70–90%), stomach, small intestine, bronchus and elsewhere: there may be multiple tumours. Clinical features include palpitations, wheezing, asthma, paroxysmal coughing, hypotension, abdominal colic, regurgitation and stenosis of the pulmonary and tricuspid valves, and skin manifestations.

The skin manifestations include: (a) episodic flushing of the face and neck, lasting at first for only a few minutes, but becoming worse in frequency, intensity and duration; eventually the face is permanently flushed, with enlarged veins, venules and capillaries, and telangiectasia (clumps of dilated vessels); (b) yellowish-brown or brown-grey patches on the forehead, wrist, back and thighs; (c) pellagra-like lesions and (d) hyperpigmentation.

Cardio-auditory syndrome. See Jervell–Lange–Nielson syndrome

Cardiorespiratory syndrome of obesity. See Pickwickian syndrome

Cardiotomy syndrome

Other name Postcardiotomy syndrome

Cardiotomy syndrome is characterized by fever and pericarditis, often associated with pleurisy or pneumonia, developing weeks or months after cardiac surgery. It may be due to an autoimmune process triggered by a viral infection. The course is benign and self-limiting.

Carotid artery syndrome

Reduction of the size of the lumen of the carotid artery, as by atherosclerosis, causes carotid insufficiency with the production of ischaemic attacks, which can last for minutes or hours. There is a motor and sensory disturbance on the opposite side of the body with amaurosis fugax (transient or partial blindness) on the side of the lesion. A hemiplegic stroke can occur.

Carotid sinus syndrome

Other names Carotid sinus reflex; pressoreceptor reflex

Stimulation of an over-sensitive carotid sinus can cause vasodilatation, slowing of the heart, a fall in blood pressure, syncope and heart block.

Carpal tunnel syndrome

In carpal tunnel syndrome tingling, burning and weakness occur in the thumb and the first and lateral half of the middle finger, with wasting of the opponens pollicis and abductor pollicis brevis muscles (i.e. the structures supplied by the median nerve) when the compression is severe. It usually occurs in the dominant hand, and the sensory disturbance is worse at night. Phalen's test is positive when flexion of the wrist produces symptoms within 1 minute. It is due to a compression of the median nerve in the carpal tunnel as a result of repeated trauma, thickening of connective tissue in hypothyroidism, acromegaly and rheumatoid arthritis, or amyloid infiltration of the transverse carpal ligament. The incidence in women is eight times greater than that in men, with a peak age of 40–50 years. It can occur in a woman in the third trimester of pregnancy owing to a general or local oedema and it then usually clears up shortly after delivery. It can also occur in women about 3 weeks after childbirth, the cause of this being unknown.

Carpenter syndrome

Other name Acrocephalosyndactyly type II

Carpenter syndrome is a congenital syndrome in which there is acrocephaly (a high pointed skull) sometimes of severe degree, premature closing of the cranial sutures, hypertelorism (wide spacing of the eyes), a flat nasal bridge and a hypoplastic mandible. Webbing of digits three and four is present; there may be abnormalities of the toes. Other features can be short neck, omphalocele, pulmonary stenosis, atrial ventricular defect or Fallot tetralogy syndrome.

Cataract-oligophrenia syndrome. See Marinesco–Sjögren syndrome

Cauda equina syndrome

Cauda equina syndrome is numbness, pain or loss of function in the legs, anaesthesia of the sacral region and sphincter disturbances due to a tumour, injury or infection involving the cauda equina. A proliferative arachnoiditis or a transverse myelitis can be due to an infection introduced in the course of spinal anaesthesia or by the use of an inappropriate drug to produce anaesthesia. It can occur in ankylosing spondylitis due to reduction in the diameter of the lumbar canal.

Cavernous sinus syndrome

Other name Foix syndrome

Cavernous sinus syndrome is characterized by paralysis of the third, fourth and sixth cranial nerves, oedema of the conjunctiva and eyelids, and proptosis (forward bulging of the eye), due to a thrombosis of the cavernous sinus. It can also be caused by aneurysm of the cavernous sinus or by invasive tumours from the sinuses and the sella turcica.

Central airways stenosis syndrome

Central airways stenosis syndrome is a stenosis of the trachea, of unknown origin but possibly the result of an infection.

Central anticholinergic syndrome

Restlessness, excitement, hallucinations and sometimes coma can be caused by anticholinergic drugs, especially in elderly patients.

Central cervical cord syndrome

Central cervical cord syndrome can follow an injury to the spinal cord by, usually, a hyperflexion injury, with blood tracking along the central canal of the cord. There is likely to be tetraplegia with the arms being more affected than the legs and with sensory loss in the arms, particularly of pain and temperature sense.
See also Cervical cord contusion syndrome

Central cord syndrome

Central cord syndrome is a painless flaccid paralysis of the arms, with urinary retention, preservation of power in the legs and preservation of dorsal column sensation in all limbs. It is due to reduction of the blood supply to the centre of the spinal cord following ossification of the posterior longitudinal ligament of the spinal column.

Central core syndrome

Central core syndrome is a familial disease of muscle in which in the majority of nerve fibres there are cores in which mitochondria are absent and the myofibrils are abnormal. The condition presents as a 'floppy infant' and is stationary or slowly progressive.

Cerebellopontine-angle tumour syndrome

A neurilemmoma or other tumour in the cerebellopontine angle can cause impairment or loss of hearing, tinnitus, paralysis of the sixth and seventh cranial nerves on the same side, vertigo, nystagmus and vomiting and ataxia due to cerebellar disturbance.

Cerebrohepatorenal syndrome. See Zellweger syndrome

Cerebro-oculo-facial-skeletal syndrome

Other name COFS syndrome

Cerebro-oculo-facial-skeletal syndrome is an autosomal recessive condition characterized by microcephaly, small jaw, flexor contractures, hypotonia, cataracts and narrowing of the palpebral fissures.

Cervical cord contusion syndrome

A fall backwards or a fall forwards onto the forehead, with a severe hyperflexion or hyperextension injury can cause tetraplegia and anaesthesia below the neck. It usually occurs in old people and especially those with cervical spondylosis. Features of the anterior cord syndrome and of the central cervical cord syndrome may be present. With incomplete lesions recovery can begin quickly, with the patient being left in the end with a mild or moderate weakness; but failure to show signs of improvement within 24 hours suggests that the prognosis is bad.

Cervical rib syndrome

Tingling and pain in the medial side of the arm and forearm, anaesthesia with coldness and cyanosis of the medial side of the palm and wasting of the small muscles of the hand are due to compression of the lower cord of the brachial plexus by a cervical rib arising from the seventh cervical vertebra. *See also* Costoclavicular syndrome and Scalenus syndrome

Cervical root syndrome

Pain in the upper outer quadrant of the breast, extending to the outer subclavicular region or to the shoulder is due to an osteophytic encroachment on a nerve exit foramen, as will be visible on an X-ray of the cervical spine.

Chediak–Higashi syndrome

Chediak–Higashi syndrome is a multisystem autosomal recessive inherited disorder (described separately by Chediak in Cuba and Higashi in Japan). Peroxidase-positive lysosomal granules are present in granulocytes and giant granules in Schwann cells and other tissues. Clinical features are oculocutaneous albinism with depigmentation of the hair, skin and retina, recurrent bacterial infections, strabismus, nystagmus and photophobia. Staphylococcal, streptococcal and fungal infections of the respiratory tract and skin occur in early childhood: later there can be fits, an enlarged liver and spleen, jaundice, enlarged hilar lymph nodes, gingivitis and pseudomembranous sloughing of the buccal mucosa. At about 5–6 years of age a progressive neuropathy is liable to involve cranial and peripheral nerves. Lymphoreticular malignancy can be a complication. Death usually occurs in childhood or the teens, and usually from an infection.

Cheiro-oral syndrome

Cheiro-oral syndrome is a sensory defect around the corner of the mouth and on the palm of the hand on the same side. It may be due to a small lesion in the contralateral post-central gyrus of the parietal lobe or to a small lesion in the thalamus. The name comes from the Greek 'cheir', which means 'hand'.

Cherry-red spot myoclonus syndrome

Other name Sialidosis

Cherry-red spot myoclonus syndrome is an autosomal recessive condition characterized by a cherry-red spot at the macula, cataracts, visual failure, myoclonus and ataxia. Skin fibroblasts show sialidase deficiency, and the urine contains large amounts of sialic acid-containing oligosaccharide.

Chiari syndrome. See Budd–Chiari syndrome

Chinese restaurant syndrome

A burning feeling in the face, a throbbing headache, light-headedness, a feeling of tightness of the jaw, neck and shoulders are due to transient arterial dilatation induced in some people by monosodium glutamate, which is used to flavour Chinese food.

Chin–sternum–heart syndrome

Chin–sternum–heart syndrome can occur when a parachute jumper with a partially opened parachute makes a hard landing upright. His chin strikes the sternum and the sternum strikes the heart. Contusion of the heart can occur. It may be asymptomatic or present with precordial pain (similar to that produced by myocardial infarction), palpitations, tachycardia, rhythm disturbances, heart murmurs and pericardial friction rub.

Chotzen syndrome

Other name Acrocephalosyndactyly type III

Acrocephaly (a tall pointed head) and craniosynostosis (premature fusion of the cranial sutures) can be associated with renal failure.

Christ–Siemens–Touraine syndrome

Other name Anhidrotic ectodermal dysplasia

Christ–Siemens–Touraine syndrome is a sex-linked recessive ectodermal-deficiency disorder, in which absence of sweat glands impairs heart regulation and causes heat intolerance. The sebaceous glands are also absent. Lacrimation can be reduced. The hair and teeth are poorly developed. Affected children may have a distinctive face with an underdeveloped maxilla and mandible, thick lips, deformed ears, prominent supraorbital ridges and a depressed bridge of the nose. Recurrent chest infections are likely. Survival to adult life can occur.

Chromosome breakage syndromes

Chromosome breakage syndromes are:
    ataxia telangiectasia
    Bloom's syndrome
    Fanconi's anaemia
They are cancer-prone syndromes in which there are thought to be defects in DNA repair.

Chronic brain syndrome

Chronic brain syndrome is any psychiatric illness believed to be due to a physical disorder of the brain.

Chronic fatigue syndrome

Other names Myalgic encephalomyelitis; Royal Free disease; postviral fatigue syndrome

Chronic fatigue syndrome is a generalized persistent or relapsing fatigue, severe enough to interfere with normal activities, associated with impairment of concentration and memory, depression, muscle and joint pain, paraesthesiae, headache and tinnitus. There may be muscle tenderness and pharyngitis. An epidemic of it among nurses in the Royal Free Hospital, London, was originally thought to be hysterical, but the condition is probably the result of a viral infection. A similar condition is known to follow toxoplasmosis and infection by the Epstein–Barr virus.

Churg–Strauss syndrome

Other name Allergic granulomatous angiitis

Churg–Strauss syndrome is an association of fever, asthma, eosinophilia with vascular and extravascular granulomas and inflammation of small arteries.

Chylomicronaemia syndrome

Other names Lipoprotein lipase deficiency; apolipoprotein C2 deficiency

Chylomicronaemia syndrome is an autosomal recessive disorder due to deficiency of either lipoprotein lipase or apolipoprotein C2 which activates lipoprotein lipase. Chylomicrons accumulate in the blood, severe hypertriglyceridaemia occurs, and macrophages are laden with fat. Clinical features are eruptive xanthomata, enlarged liver and spleen, and attacks of acute pancreatitis, due to the blocking of pancreatic capillaries by chylomicrons. Diagnosis is by (a) a positive fat deprivation diet for 3 days, which should cause an 80% reduction of plasma triglyceride and (b) lipoprotein and apolipoprotein assays.

Claude syndrome

Vascular occlusion, tumor or aneurysm involving the red nucleus in the midbrain results in oculomotor palsy with contralateral cerebellar ataxia and tremor.

Clefting syndrome

Clefting syndrome is a familial condition in which cleft palate is associated with a sunken bridge of the nose and retinal degeneration. Detachment of the retina can occur.

Click-murmur syndrome. See Prolapsed mitral valve syndrome

Clonidine withdrawal syndrome

Sudden withdrawal of clonidine hydrochloride can produce, about 20 hours later, anxiety, headache, sweating, palpitations, abdominal pains and hypertension symptoms which may last for 7–10 days.

Cloverleaf skull deformity syndrome

Cloverleaf skull deformity syndrome is characterized by a trilobed skull, exophthalmos, downward displacement of the eyes, a beaked nose and projecting jaws. It is due to an intrauterine synostosis of the coronal and lamboid sutures. Other skeletal abnormalities can be present.

Coats syndrome

In Coat syndrome telangiectasia (a small group of dilated blood vessels) of the retinal blood vessels and widespread exudation of the retina occur, most commonly in otherwise healthy boys. It can present as leukoria (a white appearance of the pupil). If untreated it can progress to total retinal detachment.

Cobb syndrome

Cobb syndrome is a haemangioma of the skin of the chest, associated with a haemangioma of a corresponding segment of the spinal meninges.

Cockayne syndrome

Cockayne syndrome is an autosomal recessive condition in which there is a defect of RNA repair. It usually presents in the 2nd year of life. Clinical features are slow physical development, short stature, sparse hair, sensorineural deafness, cataracts, blindness due to retinal degeneration, sensitivity to sunlight, thick skull bones, a bird-like facies, loss of subcutaneous fat which causes a prematurely senile appearance, and mental retardation. Other features can be microcephaly, normal-pressure hydrocephalus, and a slowly progressive peripheral neuropathy. The electrocardiogram (EEG) may show abnormalities. The thickened skull is evident on X-ray. It is not associated with an increased incidence of neoplasms.

Coeliac artery compression syndrome

Other name Median arcuate ligament syndrome

Compression of the coeliac trunk at or immediately beyond its origin from the abdominal aorta can cause abdominal pain, nausea and vomiting. The compression has been attributed to the median arcuate ligament of the diaphragm, but this does not always explain the degree of compression, which has also been attributed to fibrous tissue in the neighbourhood of the coeliac ganglion.

Coffin–Lowry syndrome

Other name Coffin–Sirus syndrome

In this familial sex-linked syndrome mental retardation is associated with coarse features, scoliosis, pigeon breast, nail defects and sometimes absence of the fifth fingers. Males can show the full syndrome; females may have only mental retardation and abnormal fingers.

COFS syndrome. See Cerebro-oculo-facial skeletal syndrome

Cogan syndrome

Other name Congenital ocular motor apraxia

Cogan syndrome is an inherited disorder in which the child is unable to move the eyes in a horizontal plane and has difficulty in following moving objects. Other eye movements are normal. The child develops a characteristic jerk of the head.

Cogan keratitis syndrome

Cogan keratitis syndrome is a non-syphilitic interstitial keratitis of the eye, associated with the vertigo, deafness and tinnitus typical of Ménière's disease.

Cohen syndrome

Cohen syndrome is an autosomal recessive inherited disorder characterized by obesity, myotonia and mental retardation but without short stature or hypogonadism.

Collet–Sicard syndrome. See Sicard syndrome

Compartmental syndrome

Compartmental syndrome is an ischaemia due to a rise of pressure within a closed fascial compartment.

See also Anterior tibial syndrome

Congenital adrenogenital syndrome

Other names Adrenogenital syndrome; congenital adrenal hyperplasia; adrenal virilism

This inherited disease may present at birth or later. It is a group of conditions in which adrenal hyperplasia is associated with a defect in the synthesis of glucocorticoids and mineralocorticoids. The regulation of adrenocorticotrophic hormone (ACTH) by negative feedbacks is interfered with and as a result the secretion of ACTH by the pituitary is unchecked. The highest incidence – 2.0 per 1000 live births – is in the Inuit (Eskimos). Clinical features are virilization, thickening and coarsening of the skin, acne, excessive growth of bushy hair, hyperpigmentation of the skin of the axillae, breasts, perianal region and external genitalia, hypotension, sodium retention and hypokalaemia. Male infants show pseudo-hermaphroditism (they look like females) and boys show a premature development of pubic and axillary hair, male-type alopecia of the scalp, enlargement of the penis and increased folding of the scrotal skin. Female infants show masculinization. Women have primary amenorrhoea, an enlarged clitoris, a failure of breast development, severe acne, excess hair and increased muscular development. Adult men show little change in normal appearance and development.

Congenital laryngeal stridor syndrome

Congenital laryngeal stridor syndrome is a stridor on inspiration, developing with the first few days or weeks of life and due usually to loose aryepiglottic folds which collapse on inspiration. There may be a deformity of the larynx or epiglottis. The stridor is made worse by crying but gradually lessens and disappears within 12–18 months.

Congenital nephrotic syndrome

Other names Finnish type disease; microcytic disease

Congenital nephrotic syndrome is an autosomal recessive inherited disorder presenting at birth or shortly afterwards. Clinical features are severe proteinuria, failure to thrive, malnutrition and death likely from infection.

See also Nephrotic syndrome

Congenital rubella syndrome. See Rubella syndrome

Conn syndrome

Other name Primary hyperaldosteronism

The excess of aldosterone is produced by an adrenal cortical adenoma or by hyperplasia of the zona granulosa of the adrenal glands. Sodium and water are retained by the kidney. Clinical features are hypertension, cardiomyopathy, retinopathy, polyuria, muscle weakness, intermittent paralysis, cardiac arrhythmias, paraesthesiae, tetany-like symptoms and psychiatric disturbances.

Conradi syndrome

Other name Chondrodystrophy calcificans

Conradi syndrome is a familial (dominant) or sporadic syndrome characterized by short stature, chondrodystrophy with characteristic punctate calcification of the epiphyses (visible on X-ray) and scaling of the skin, which clears up during the 1st year of life and leaves behind atrophic areas and cicatrical alopecia. Renal disease, congenital heart disease and mental retardation can be present.

Contiguous gene syndromes

This is a group of disorders in which there are small chromosomal abnormalities and there are recurrent and recognizable patterns of physical malformations, usually associated with mental retardation. They are:

Beckwith–Wiedemann syndrome
Di George syndrome
Haemoglobin H-mental retardation
Lancer–Gideon syndrome
Miller–Dieker syndrome
Prader–Willi syndrome
Retinoblastoma
Wilms tumour

Coracoid impingement syndrome. See Rotator cuff impingement syndrome

Cornelia de Lange syndrome

Other name De Lange syndrome

Cornelia de Lange syndrome is an autosomal recessive inherited disorder characterized by a lobster-claw deformity of the hands, short stature, microcephaly, cleft lip and palate, optic atrophy, an upturned nose, bushy eyebrows, hirsutism, a low hair-line, a beaked upper lip and a notched lower lip, marbled skin, webbed toes, hypoplastic nipples, a failure to thrive and mental retardation.

Corticosteroid withdrawal syndrome

Other name Steroid withdrawal syndrome

Sudden withdrawal of corticosteroids can induce mild and severe symptoms. Mild ones are conjunctivitis, rhinitis, painful itchy nodules, painful muscles and joints, fatigue, weakness, loss of appetite and a low-grade fever. More serious are acute adrenal insufficiency and hypotension.

Costen syndrome

Pain in the temporomandibular joint is due to malocclusion (apposing teeth are not properly related when the mouth is closed) or to arthritis of the joint as part of a generalized arthritis such as rheumatoid arthritis. There can be severe aching pain which is increased by chewing.

Costochondral junction syndrome. See Tietze syndrome

Costoclavicular syndrome

Compression of the lower cord of the brachial plexus between the clavicle and the first rib causes symptoms and signs similar to those of the cervical rib syndrome.

Cough syndrome

Loss of consciousness is induced by coughing. The electrocardiogram may show a cough-induced paroxysmal arterioventricular block with ventricular asystole. Severe prolonged coughing may cause a lowered cerebral perfusion pressure, which leads to increased intrathoracic pressure with reduction of cardiac output and impairment of cerebral venous return via the jugular veins.

Couvade syndrome

Couvade syndrome is the physical and emotional health problems experienced by a man during his partner's pregnancy and in the immediate postpartum period. Men particularly likely to develop it have had a health problem during the previous year. Also likely to develop it are men with low incomes, men with previous children, men with a highly emotional interest in the pregnancy, men with economic and personal stresses and men from an ethnic minority. Common complaints are of nausea, vomiting and abdominal pain.

Cowden syndrome. See Multiple hamartoma syndrome

Cracked tooth syndrome

The patient with a cracked tooth complains of pain on biting and of discomfort or pain produced by hot or cold drinks or food. Mobility of the fragments can occur. Pulpitis and periodontal abscess can be complications.

Crain syndrome

Crain syndrome is a recurrent and progressive arthritis of the interphalangeal joints which occurs usually in middle-aged women and is not attributable to rheumatoid arthritis.

Craniodiaphyseal dysplasia syndrome

Craniodiaphyseal dysplasia syndrome is characterized by hyperostosis and sclerosis, especially of the skull and facial bones; involvement of the cranial foramina can cause paralysis of cranial nerves, with pressure on the optic and auditory nerves causing blindness and deafness. Other features are growth retardation, convulsions and mental retardation.

CREST syndrome

CREST syndrome is a multisystem syndrome similar to systemic sclerosis but running a slower course and characterized by:

- C – calcification, subcutaneous nodular
- R – Raynaud syndrome
- E – esophageal dysfunction
- S – sclerodactyly (scleroderma of the fingers and toes)
- T – telangiectasia (angiomas formed by dilated capillaries), most common on the hands and feet.

Cri-du-chat syndrome

Deletion of the short arm of chromosome 5 causes severe mental retardation, deformity of the larynx (a coarse unpleasant miaow-like sound being produced), microcephaly, hypertelorism (wide spacing of the eyes), prominent ears and short stature.

Crigler–Najjar syndrome

In this autosomal recessive condition, absence of the hepatic enzyme glucuronyl transferase causes a severe jaundice, an excess of bilirubin in the blood, kernicterus (degeneration of the basal ganglia) and severe disorders of the central nervous system. If the absence of the enzyme is total (type I), the condition rapidly causes death; if it is partial (type II), the patient can survive.

Cronkhite–Canada syndrome. See Canada–Cronkhite syndrome

Crossed brainstem syndromes. See Brainstem syndromes

Cross–McKusick–Breen syndrome

Other names Cross syndrome; oculocerebral-hypopigmentation syndrome

Cross–McKusick–Breen syndrome is an autosomal recessive inherited disorder characterized by a reduction of pigment in the skin and eyes, microphthalmia, nystagmus, cloudy corneas, writhing movements of the arms and legs, a highly-pitched cry, gingival fibromatosis and severely retarded physical and mental development. Malignant tumours of the skin can be a complication.

Crouzon syndrome

Other name Craniofacial dysostosis

Crouzon syndrome is an autosomal dominant condition characterized by premature closure of the cranial sutures, an abnormally shaped head, hypertelorism (wide spacing of the eyes), a beaked nose and hypoplasia of the maxilla. The skull deformity may be a brachycephaly, scaphocephaly, trigonocephaly (triangular shape due to a midline angulation of the frontal bone) or cloverleaf. Other features can be strabismus, nystagmus and exophthalmos. The palate is highly arched and can be cleft. There may be malocclusion of the teeth. Increased intracranial pressure can occur.

Crush syndrome

Crush syndrome is oliguria, oedema and renal failure following the crush of a large muscle mass or other large part of the body.

Cubital tunnel syndrome

Compression of the ulnar nerve in the cubital tunnel at the elbow can cause numbness and pain in the skin supplied by the nerve and weakness of the muscles it supplies.

Cushing syndrome

The causes of Cushing syndrome are an excess of adrenocorticotrophic hormone (ACTH) produced by adrenal hyperplasia, adrenal adenoma or adrenal carcinoma, or a pituitary adenoma, or ectopic production of ACTH from a non-pituitary carcinoma. It can also be caused by treatment with corticosteroids. Clinical features are a 'buffalo hump' (an excessive deposit of fat over the clavicles and back of the neck), abdominal obesity, cutaneous striae, purpura, a florid complexion, hirsutism, a 'moon-shaped' face, wasted limbs, weakness and fatiguability, oedema, acne, amenorrhoea, osteoporosis (and hence pathological fractures), and eosinophilia. Children with it have stunted growth. Diabetes mellitus can be a complication. A reduction in height can be due to osteoporosis and compression fractures of the vertebrae.

Cyriax syndrome

Cyriax syndrome is pain caused by pressure on intercostal nerves by malformations of ribs eight to ten or an excessive mobility of their forward ends.

D

Dancing eyes syndrome

Dancing eyes syndrome is an eye movement disorder in which there are rapid and random conjugate movements of the eyes. It can occur in a patient with a neuroblastoma or a carcinoma, and can be associated with myoclonus in the limbs in brainstem encephalitis.

Dandy–Walker syndrome

Dandy–Walker syndrome is a hydrocephalus in a neonate due to a failure of development of the foramina of Luschka and Magendie (the foramina in the roof of the fourth ventricle of the brain). Because of this failure, the cerebrospinal fluid cannot pass into the subarachnoid space and in consequence accumulates in the ventricles.

Dapsone syndrome

Treatment with dapsone in doses of 100–300 mg daily can cause muscle and joint pain, urticaria, cough, enlarged lymph nodes and an atypical lymphocytosis with a negative Paul Bunnell test.

Dead hand syndrome. See Vibration syndrome

Debré–de Toni–Fanconi syndrome. See Fanconi syndrome

Debré–Semelaigne syndrome

Debré–Semelaigne syndrome is a pseudohypertrophy of muscles occurring in hypothyroidism. The enlarged muscles are weak and slow to contract and relax.

De Clérambault syndrome

The patient is usually a woman. She becomes deluded that a certain man is in love with her. The man is usually older and of higher social status. The man, who has done nothing to stimulate or encourage such a belief, is at first unaware of it but is later likely to be embarrassed by telephone calls, letters and amorous advances.

Defibrination syndrome

Other name Disseminated intravascular coagulation (DIC)

Defibrination syndrome is characterized by shock, haemorrhage and renal failure following activation of the blood coagulation mechanism within the circulation. Among the conditions in which it can occur are septicaemia, viral infections, malaria, incompatible blood transfusion, trauma and snake bites. Fibrin is deposited within the small blood vessels and fibrin/fibrinogen split products appear to excessive amounts in the blood and urine. These split products increase the haemorrhagic tendency and promote hypotension. Red blood cells are destroyed as they pass through a fibrin web in the blood vessels. Haemorrhages into the skin, from mucous membranes and from the genital tract, can occur and haematomas develop at suture or injection sites.

Déjerine–Roussy syndrome. See Thalamic syndrome

De Lange syndrome. See Cornelia de Lange syndrome

Del Castillo syndrome. See Sertoli cell only syndrome

Demarquay syndrome. See Lip pit syndrome

Denial syndrome

Denial syndrome is a refusal to admit the existence of severe physical disease or disability, usually in the case of a brain-damaged patient.

De Sanctis–Cacchione syndrome

De Sanctis–Cacchione syndrome is a recessive inherited condition with degeneration of cerebral and cerebellar neurons. Clinical features can include microcephaly, short stature, gonadal dysplasia, xeroderma pigmentosa, mental retardation, a progressive neurological and mental deterioration, with spasticity, choreoathetosis, ataxia and shortening of the Achilles tendon.

Dhat syndrome

Dhat syndrome is a culture-associated male sex neurosis of men of the Indian subcontinent or from it. The man complains of passing 'dhat', a whitish substance, in the urine, which however is usually normal in appearance. He believes that the substance is semen and that with it he is losing his virility. He complains of aching, bodily weakness, mental exhaustion and depression.

DIDMOAD syndrome

Other name Wolfram syndrome

DIDMOAD syndrome is an association of:

DI – diabetes insipidus
DM – diabetes mellitus
OA – optical atrophy
D – deafness

Diencephalic syndrome of infancy

Diencephalic syndrome of infancy is characterized by loss of subcutaneous fat, hypoglycaemia, hypotension and pallor of the skin in an infant. It is usually due to a tumour involving the anterior hypothalamus of the brain.

Di George syndrome

Other name Third and fourth pharyngeal pouch syndrome

Di George syndrome is one of the contiguous gene syndromes. In it there is a small deletion from chromosome 22, detectable by gene mapping or the use of restriction fragment length polymorphism. The parathyroid glands are absent, the thymus is absent or aplastic and a cell deficiency occurs during the first 3 months of life. Clinical features include severe chronic infections (to which resistance is low), deformities of the ears, nose and mouth, abnormalities of the great vessels, obstruction of the aortic arch, hypoparathyroidism, tetany and cardiac failure.

Di Guglielmo syndrome

Other name Acute erythroleukaemia

In Di Guglielmo syndrome, of unknown origin, enormous numbers of nucleated red cells appear in the bone marrow and blood. It may be a variant of acute myeloblastic leukaemia.

Disc syndrome

Low back pain, pain in the thigh, sometimes with wasting of the thigh and loss of knee and ankle jerks are due to pressure on nerve roots by a slipped intervertebral disc.

Disconnection syndrome

Disconnection syndrome is a term applied to several disorders in which one part of the brain is disconnected from another, such as happens when one hemisphere is disconnected from the other by section of the corpus callosum.

See also Alexia without agraphia syndrome

Disequilibrium syndrome

Headache, nausea and muscular cramps, followed by agitation, fits, delirium and coma can occur during rapid dialysis in the early stage of a dialysis programme. It is thought to be due to a shift of water into the brain, producing symptoms similar to those produced by water intoxication.

Disialotransferrin developmental syndrome

Disialotransferrin developmental syndrome is characterized by failure to thrive in infancy, hypotonia, developmental delay, joint restriction, mild non-progressive liver disease, cerebellar hypoplasia, retinal dystrophy, and pericardial effusion. The syndrome resembles olivopontocerebellar atrophy with neonatal onset.

Distichia syndrome

Distichia syndrome is a familial dominant syndrome in which distichia (a double row of eyelashes on one lid with one or both rows turned inwards onto the eyeball) is associated with lymphoedema of the legs and sometimes with vertebral defects.

Donohue syndrome

Other name Leprechaunism

Donohue syndrome is a familial (recessive) syndrome characterized by a broad nose, hypertelorism (wide spacing of the eyes), low-set large ears, short stature, bone dystrophy, large penis in males, ovarian cyst in females, sexual precocity and mental retardation.

A leprechaun is an ugly but friendly little spirit who helps Irish housewives with their work.

Dorsal root ganglion syndrome

Dorsal root ganglion syndrome is characterized by severe pain in the arm following a cervical hyperflexion or hyperextension injury. The pain is made worse by extension or flexion of the head. There is usually no sensory loss. It is thought to be due to contusion and haemorrhage into and around the dorsal root ganglia in the neck.

Down syndrome

Other name Trisomy 21 syndrome

The presence of three chromosomes number 21 causes severe mental retardation (IQ usually under 50) and characteristic physical abnormalities. The only known aetiological factor is increased maternal age. The risk of a Down syndrome per 1000 live births is 0.7 for a woman under 30 years of age: for a woman of 40–44 years it is 13.1 per 1000 live births, and for a woman over 45 it is 34.6 per 1000 live births. However, because young women have more babies than older women, most Down syndrome babies are born to young mothers – 51% to mothers under 30 years and 72% to mothers under 35 years.

Physical features include short stature, a round small head, a short neck, a mongoloid slant of the eyes, an epicanthic fold of the eyelids, a fissured and enlarging tongue, a transverse palmar crease, a rough skin and obesity in older patients, and muscle hypotonia. Congenital heart disease occurs in about 50% of patients and is a major cause of morbidity and mortality: the defects can be endocardial cushion defects, septal defects, Fallot's tetralogy and a patent ductus arteriosus. Gastrointestinal abnormalities include pyloric stenosis, duodenal atresia or stenosis and Hirschsprung's disease. Pulmonary infection is common. Infantile spasms and myoclonic seizures can occur. Tonsillar hypertrophy can cause obstructive sleep apnoea. There may be defects of the cervical spine, atlantoaxial subluxation can cause a stiff neck, and an atlantoaxial dislocation can occur and be fatal. Some patients have alopecia areata. There is an increased incidence over the usual of acute lymphoblastic leukaemia. Over the age of 30 years, there is a high incidence of orofacial dyskinesia (abnormal movements of the face and mouth). Patients who survive into the fourth and fifth decades develop the pathological changes of Alzheimer's disease in the brain.

Some patients show mosaicism – a mixture of normal and trisomic cell lines – and in them the IQ can be in the 70s and the physical abnormalities may not be so marked.

It can be diagnosed *in utero* by chorion villous biopsy at 11 weeks (which carries a risk of abortion of 2–3%) or amniocentesis at 16 weeks (which carries a risk of abortion of 1–2%). Tests of maternal blood which are being developed and by which Down syndrome can be detected in 80%

of cases are (a) for raised activity level of urea-resistant neutrophil alkaline phosphatase (UR-NAP), an enzyme found in white blood cells, and (b) a 'triple marker test' of oestriol, human chorionic gonadotrophin and α-fetoprotein.

Dressler syndrome. See Postmyocardial infarction syndrome

Drug abuse syndromes

Abused drugs usually have a direct effect on the central nervous system. The drug abuser is likely to have unexplained episodes or altered behaviour or consciousness and neurological complications.

Dry eye syndrome. See Stevens–Johnson syndrome

Duane syndrome

Duane syndrome is a genetically determined, usually autosomal recessive, condition of deficient horizontal ocular movements and strabismus. The lateral rectus muscle is usually more affected that the medial rectus muscle. Attempted adduction causes retraction of the globe and narrowing of the palpebral fissure. It was thought to be due to fibrosis of the muscles, but electromyographic investigation suggests that it may be partly a disorder of innervation.

Dubin–Johnson syndrome

Other name Chronic idiopathic jaundice

Dubin–Johnson syndrome is a familial benign jaundice due to a defective excretion by the liver of bilirubin and other organic ions. The hepatic cells show pathognomic coarse granules. As steroid metabolism is blocked and ovarian steroids undergo metabolism in the liver, oral contraceptives can be a risk.

Dubowitz syndrome

Dubowitz syndrome is an autosomal recessive inherited disorder characterized by low birth weight, short stature, a high sloping forehead, a broad nasal bridge, sparse fine hair, sometimes eczema and mental retardation.

Dumping syndrome

Dumping syndrome is characterized by postprandial nausea, flushing, sweating, palpitations, abdominal fullness, borborygmi and sometimes diarrhoea, occurring after partial gastrectomy. An attack lasts for about 30 minutes. An *early form* occurs during or immediately after a meal: it is due to the rapid transfer of fluid into the small intestine and an osmotic shift of fluid into the intestine with the production of hypotension. A *later form* occurs 2 hours or more after a meal and may be due to hypoglycaemia following a rapid production of insulin. The patient may have a history of allergy or of psychological instability.

Dyggve syndrome

Other name Dyggve–Melchior–Claussen syndrome

Dyggve syndrome is an autosomal recessive condition characterized by short stature, sternal bulging, flattened vertebral bodies, clawed fingers and mental retardation.

Dysarthria-clumsy hand syndrome

Dysarthria-clumsy hand syndrome is one of the 'lacunar syndromes' in which lacunae (small spaces) appear in the brain. In this syndrome lacunae are present in the genu and anterior limb of the internal capsule. The clinical features are severe dysarthria (imperfect articulation), facial palsy and paralysis of the tongue, associated with clumsiness and slight weakness of the hand.

Dysmenic syndrome

Dysmenic syndrome is a disorder of memory due to cerebral degeneration in which new information is promptly forgotten and old information well remembered beyond the degree that can be considered normal in old age.

Dysplastic naevus syndrome. See Familial atypical multiple mole-melanoma syndrome

E

Eagle–Barrett syndrome. See Prune belly syndrome

Easy bruising syndrome

Easy bruising syndrome is a common condition, usually of women in whom bruises appear spontaneously or after minimal trauma. Laboratory tests are normal. The condition is probably due to an increased fragility of capillaries. Patients should be advised to avoid aspirin, which may make the condition worse.

Eaton–Lambert syndrome

Other name Myasthenic syndrome

Eaton–Lambert syndrome is a disorder of neuromuscular transmission due to a reduction of acetylcholine release at the motor endplate, presumed to be due to impaired acetylcholine esterase activity. It is most common in adults over the age of 40 years and more common in men than in women, but incidence is about equal when a bronchial carcinoma is not present. Characteristic features are weakness and fatiguability in the proximal muscles of the limbs (more commonly in the arms than in the legs), weak or absent tendon reflexes, impotence, difficulties in micturition, dry mouth and constipation. A small-cell carcinoma of the lung is commonly present. Associated diseases are in adults hyperthyroidism and hypothyroidism and in children systemic lupus erythematosus, leukaemia, neuroblastoma and rheumatoid arthritis.

Ectopic corticotrophin syndrome

Excessive corticotrophin secretion by various tumours – oat-cell bronchial carcinoma, thymoma, phaeochromocytoma, C-cell tumour – causes a rapidly developing Cushing syndrome with fluid retention, oedema, hypertension, hypokalaemia, muscle weakness and, less commonly, facial plethora and obesity. Plasma and urinary cortisol and plasma corticotrophin levels are raised.

Ectopic vasopressin syndrome

Excess vasopressin (antidiuretic hormone) produced by a tumour – usually an oat-cell bronchial carcinoma – causes water retention, nausea, vomiting, headache and confusion: coma can be followed by death. Serum sodium levels are low, sometimes as low as 110 mmol/l.

Edwards syndrome

Other name Trisomy 18 syndrome

Trisomy 18 causes multiple abnormalities: mental retardation, an abnormally shaped skull, low-set abnormal ears, a small mandible, congenital heart disease of various kinds, abnormal fingers, diaphragmatic hernia, inguinal hernia, adducted hips, enlarged external genitalia, rocker-bottom feet and Meckel's diverticulum.

EEC syndrome

EEC syndrome is an autosomal dominant inherited condition characterized by:

E – ectrodactyly (congenital absence of all or part of a digit)
E – ectodermal dysplasia
C – cleft lip and palate.

Associated conditions are alopecia, lacrimal duct stenosis, malformed teeth and renal abnormalities.

Effort syndrome

Effort syndrome is an anxiety state concentrated on the efficiency of the heart and circulation. The patient becomes increasingly conscious of his heart beat and respiration, which are further increased by his anxiety.

Ehlers–Danlos syndrome

Other name Cutis hyperplastica

Ehlers–Danlos syndrome is an inherited form of collagen abnormality of which eleven different variants have been described. It can be inherited as an autosomal dominant, an autosomal recessive or an X-linked recessive. It is characterized by hyperelasticity of the skin, which is loose and thickened, hyperextensibility and subluxation of joints due to lax capsules, and impaired wound healing with the production of coarse scars. Angioid streaks are present in the fundi of the eyes and retinal haemorrhages can occur. The skin, veins and tracheal mucosa are fragile. Bleeding can occur from the gastrointestinal tract, the urinary tract and the skin after minor injury. Spontaneous pneumothorax can occur. The collagen in the arterial walls can be affected and aneurysms can occur and rupture spontaneously. Hypertension can be present and the pulses in the extremities can be absent or weak because of the hyperelasticity of the arteries. Other features can be pseudoxanthoma elasticum, blue sclerae, subcutaneous calcification following trauma, and infarction of the stomach.

Eisenmenger syndrome

Eisenmenger syndrome was originally used to describe a ventricular septal defect with pulmonary hypertension and is now used to describe any left-to-right shunt lesion with pulmonary hypertension.

Ekbom syndrome. See Restless legs syndrome

Elbow tunnel syndrome

Elbow tunnel syndrome is due to an entrapment of the ulnar nerve in the cubital fossa with the loss of sensation in the medial one and a half fingers, paralysis and wasting of hypothenar, interossei and medial two lumbrical muscles.

Ellis–van Creveld syndrome

Other name Chondro-ectodermal dysplasia

Ellis–van Creveld syndrome is an autosomal recessive disorder character-ized by short limbs, a long narrow thorax, polydactyly, hypoplastic nails and teeth, and congenital heart defects such as atrial and ventricular defects and cleft mitral valve. Erupted teeth can be present at birth. Respiratory distress can be due to deficiency of tracheal and bronchial cartilage.

Elpenor syndrome

Elpenor syndrome is characterized by disorientation and behaviour disor-der on awakening from an alcoholic stupor or drug-induced sleep. It is named after Elpenor in *The Odyssey* who, 'heavy with wine', was sleeping on top of a flat roof and when he was awakened suddenly he did not appreciate where he was, fell off the roof and broke his neck – which should be a warning to anyone not to go to sleep on the top of a roof when one has had too much to drink.

EMG syndrome

EMG syndrome is a congenital condition characterized by:

E – exomphalos
M – macroglossia
G – gigantism

Hypoglycaemia can occur in the early days of life.

Empty sella syndrome

Hypopituitarism is associated with an enlarged pituitary fossa and an extension into it of the subarachnoid space, with cerebrospinal fluid in it. The pituitary gland is flattened against the bottom of the fossa which on X-ray appears to be empty. It can occur idiopathically or follow surgery or irradiation of a pituitary tumour.

Eosinophilia-myalgia syndrome

Eosinophilia-myalgia syndrome is associated with taking L-tryptophan, an antidepressive drug, but how the syndrome is caused is uncertain: it has been attributed to a contaminant of the tryptophan or it may occur in a susceptible compromised patient. Clinical features include severe eosinophilia, a severe and often incapacitating myalgia, arthralgia, interstitial lung disease, cardiac arrhythmias, sclerodermiform thickening of the skin, rashes, fatigue, dyspnoea and cough. The absolute eosinophilia count usually exceeds 2000 cells/mm^3. Myocarditis and a potentially fatal ascending polyneuropathy can occur.

Euthyroid sick syndromes

Three syndromes are classified under this term. In them there are abnormalities in circulating thyroid hormone levels in non-thyroidal illnesses.

Low T_3 syndrome
In this syndrome there is a combination of subnormal T_3 (triiodothyronine) with normal T_4 (thyroxine) in a clinically euthyroid patient. It can be present in 70–75% of hospitalized patients suffering from liver disease, kidney failure, congestive heart failure, neoplasms, fevers and burns. It is also found in calorie-deprivation states and after major surgery, and it can be due to some drugs – dexamethasone, amidarone, high doses of propranolol and prophythiouracil – and some oral cholecystography dyes.

Low T_3–T_4 syndrome
A patient in this state has a low serum concentration of total T_3 and T_4 in a

non-thyroidal illness. It is found in severely ill patients, and about 50% of patients admitted into an intensive care unit may show it. Despite the low serum T_3 and T_4 levels the patients do not appear hypothyroidal.

High T_4 syndrome
This is less common than the other two syndromes. In it there is a high level of serum T_4 in non-thyroidal illness. It is almost exclusively found in elderly sick patients; it can be due to taking propranolol in high doses.

Evans syndrome

Evans syndrome is an autoimmune (idiopathic) thrombocytopenic purpura associated with autoimmune haemolytic anaemia.

Expanded and activated melanocyte syndrome. See Familial atypical multiple mole-melanoma syndrome

Exploding head syndrome

Exploding head syndrome is a terrifying sense of an explosive noise in the head experienced usually in the twilight stage of sleep. Associated symptoms are varied. The aetiology is unknown. It appears to be benign, and intensive investigations and treatment are not indicated.

Eye-foot syndrome

Eye-foot syndrome is retinopathy and gangrene of the foot in a patient with diabetes mellitus. The prognosis for sight, limb and life is bad.

F

Fabry syndrome

Other names Anderson–Fabry syndrome; angiokeratoma corporis diffusum

Fabry syndrome is an X-linked recessive disease in which deficiency of the enzyme α-galactosidase causes the deposition of neutral glycophingolipids in tissues and fluids. Clinical features in many systems occur. (a) Peripheral neuropathy occurs with painful crises ('Fabry crises') of burning agonizing pain in the hands and feet, radiating elsewhere and lasting for minutes or days; the pain can increase or decrease in frequency and intensity with age. Between attacks, unpleasant paraesthesia is present in the hands and feet, and attacks of pain can occur in the abdomen and flanks. (b) Dark-red to bluish-red purpura-like spots appear on the lower part of the trunk, buttocks and thighs. (c) Cardiac involvement is shown by anginal pain, myocardial ischaemia, mitral insufficiency, enlargement of the heart and congestive heart failure. The EEG shows abnormalities. (d) Involvement of the cerebral arteries causes cerebral thromboses and cerebral haemorrhage and cerebral degeneration, with the production of mental deterioration and personality changes. (e) Involvement of the eyes can cause cataracts and vascular lesions of the conjunctiva and retina. (f) Involvement of the kidneys interferes with renal function and leads to death in early adult life from chronic renal failure. (g) Involvement of other organs can cause chronic bronchitis, pulmonary function deterioration, lymphoedema of the legs, diarrhoea, retarded growth and puberty, skeletal abnormalities, anaemia, fatigue and weakness.

Prenatal diagnosis can be made by assay of α-galactosidase A activity in chorionic villi or cultured amniotic cells obtained by amniocentesis.

Facet syndrome

Facet syndrome is an arthritis of the articular facets of the spinal column, mainly in the lumbar region. Clinical features are stiffness and back pain. The pain, which is described as 'locking', is relieved in some positions and increased in others.

Fahr syndrome

Other name Basal ganglia calcification

Rigidity, extrapyramidal disturbances, choreic and dystonic movements and dementia are due to calcification in the basal ganglia. It can occur in hyperparathyroidism and pseudohypoparathyroidism and, in association with cerebellar calcification, it can occur as a familial autosomal dominant inherited condition.

Failure to thrive syndrome

Other names Marasmus; anaclitic depression

Failure to thrive syndrome is a syndrome of early childhood characterized by failure to grow at a normal rate, a wasted body, thin arms and legs, vomiting, poor appetite, dark circles round the eyes, diarrhoea or constipation, listlessness, and unhappiness. It can be due to parental rejection or neglect and a sign of child abuse. Other causes are inadequate food (as in a famine), malabsorption, chronic infection, metabolic or endocrine defect, or a severe congenital abnormality. The term 'anaclitic depression' describes the miserable appearance of the child (anaclisis – dependence on the mother for love, food and care).

Fallot's tetralogy syndrome

Fallot's tetralogy syndrome is a congenital disorder of the heart consisting of a ventricular septal defect, narrowing of the right ventricular outflow or stenosis of the pulmonary artery, overriding of dextroposition of the aorta, and right ventricular hypertrophy. It forms about 10% of all forms of congenital heart disease. Clinical features are cyanosis from birth or developing in the first year of life, retarded growth and physical development, dyspnoea on exertion, clubbing of the fingers and toes, and polycythaemia. The child has a characteristic squatting position when resting after exertion. A right ventricular impulse and thrill may be felt along the left border of the sternum. On auscultation the second heart sound is single and the pulmonic component rarely heard; a mid-systolic murmur is usually present over the base of the heart.

Familial amyloidotic syndrome

In familial amyloidotic syndrome there is an accumulation of an amyloid-like substance in the peripheral nervous system with amyloid fibrils deposited in the peripheral nerves, kidneys and heart. Clinical features are a polyneuropathy with distal loss of sensation and symptoms of autonomic function disorder: postural hypotension, gastrointestinal dysfunction, abnormal sweating and impotence. It is the result of a single amino acid substitution in transthyretin (a protein formerly known as pre-albumin).

Familial atypical multiple mole-melanoma syndrome

Other names Dysplastic naevus syndrome; large atypical mole syndrome; expanded and activated melanocyte syndrome; B–K mole syndrome

Familial atypical multiple mole-melanoma syndrome is an autosomal dominant form of cutaneous melanoma. Dysplastic naevi start to appear in childhood and continue to appear into adult life; puberty and pregnancy can stimulate their appearance. They appear mainly on the back and trunk. They are usually 5–10 mm in diameter, pink to brown in colour and with an irregular outline. They can develop into malignant melanomas, and death can be due to metastases from the melanomas. There may be patches of hyperpigmented skin.

Fanconi syndrome

Other names Renal tubular acidosis; Debré–de Toni–Fanconi syndrome

In this hereditary disorder of the proximal renal tubule there is a defect in the reabsorption of glucose, amino acids, phosphate and potassium. Loss of calcium and phosphate causes hypoglycaemia and hypophosphataemia. Calcium is withdrawn from bone, causing renal rickets. Nephrocalcinosis (a deposit of calcium in the kidney and renal stone formation) can occur. Other features can be short stature, microcephaly, mental retardation, abnormalities of the radius, a reduced number of carpal bones, hypoplasia or aplasia of the thumb, absent radial pulse, hypoplastic bone marrow, congenital heart disease, hyperpigmentation of the skin, weakness, congenital dislocation of the hip, renal malformations and gradual liver failure with death likely to occur before the age of 10 years.

The syndrome can appear in the 30s and 40s without any apparent precipitating cause.

Fanconi pancytopenia syndrome

Other names Congenital aplastic anaemia with developmental abnormalities; familial constitutional panmyelocytopathy

Fanconi pancytopenia syndrome is an association of multiple congenital abnormalities: short stature, small external genitalia, patchy melanotic pigmentation of the skin, squint, nystagmus, deformities of the ears, deafness, anomalies of long bones, congenital dislocation of the hip, absent radius, abnormal or absent thumbs, and mental retardation. There is a degree of immunodeficiency, with which can be associated a squamous cell carcinoma of the mouth. The aplastic anaemia may not appear before 4 or 5 years of age. Chromosomal abnormalities may be present. Leukaemia is a complication. Transmission seems to be by an autosomal recessive gene of variable penetrance; sporadic cases can occur.

Farber syndrome

Other name Disseminated lipogranulomatosis

Farber syndrome is a mucopolysaccaride disorder characterized by peri-articular swellings, ankylosis, hypochromic anaemia, laryngeal granulomas (which can cause hoarseness), a liability to recurrent infections, and cardiac and renal failure.

Fat embolism syndrome

Fat embolism syndrome arises from the effects of multiple small emboli which are found in traumatized tissue, especially the fracture of a long bone, and block small arterioles and capillaries. Clinical features include petechiae (which appear in crops 2 or 3 days after the injury), dyspnoea, pulmonary oedema, cyanosis, a cough with or without haemoptysis, tachycardia, fever, jaundice, microscopic haematuria, restlessness, irritability, confusion and coma. The syndrome may appear as a failure to regain consciousness after orthopaedic surgery under a general anaesthetic. About 25% of patients have a patent foramen ovale. In severe cases with multiple fractures, death (usually from respiratory failure) can occur within 24 hours.

Felty syndrome

Other name Hypersplenism

In Felty syndrome rheumatoid arthritis is associated with an enlarged spleen, leukopenia, thrombocytopenia and anaemia. Other features can be weight loss, recurrent infections, pigmentation of the skin, enlarged liver, moderate lymph node enlargement, ulceration of the skin, peripheral neuropathy, carpal tunnel syndrome, arteritis, Raynaud syndrome and scleritis.

Fertile eunuch syndrome

Other name Isolated luteinizing hormone (LH) deficiency

Luteinizing hormone (LH) deficiency in the male causes a reduced secretion of testosterone. In fertile eunuch syndrome, enough testosterone is produced to maintain spermatogenesis, but not enough to produce secondary male sexual characteristics.

Fetal alcoholic syndrome

Fetal alcoholic syndrome is due to excessive drinking of alcohol by a pregnant woman. It is rare in Great Britain but it is a risk for alcoholic women who do not reduce their alcohol consumption during pregnancy. The child may show fetal growth retardation, cardiac defects (especially septal defects and Fallot's tetralogy), maxillary hypoplasia, prominent lower jaw and forehead, small palpebral fissures, small eyes, unilateral ptosis, growth retardation, mental retardation and abnormal neurobehavioural development.

Fetal smoking syndrome

Smoking by a pregnant woman can cause intrauterine growth retardation, fetal hypoxia, placental abruption, miscarriage, premature rupture of membranes in labour, premature delivery, low Apgar scores (a method of assessing and recording a neonate's skin colour, muscle tone, respiratory effort, heart rate and response to stimulus at 1, 5 and 10 minutes after birth), which can be associated with increased perinatal mortality, respiratory infections and an increased risk of sudden infant death syndrome.

Fibromyalgia syndrome

Other name Fibrositis syndrome

Fibromyalgia syndrome is characterized by chronic generalized aches and pain, stiffness and multiple 'trigger points' of hypersensitivity to pressure. Other features can be chronic headache, pain in the neck and shoulders, sleep disturbance, Raynaud syndrome and, in about 50% of cases, irritable bowel syndrome.

First and second arch syndrome. See Pierre Robin syndrome

Fish odour syndrome

Other name Trimethylaminuria

Trimethylamine is found in food in various forms, such as choline and lecithin, in liver, kidneys, eggs, soya beans, marine fish and mayonnaise. Normally it is broken down by hepatic enzymes into an odourless substance N-oxide, which is excreted in the breath, sweat and urine. People with fish odour syndrome probably have a deficiency of one of the enzymes which break down trimethylamine. They excrete the trimethylamine in their breath, sweat and urine and its rotten fish smell is apparent to others but not to them. The smell can be reduced by reducing the intake of choline-high and lecithin-high foods.

Fish tank syndrome

Other name Fish tank granuloma

Granulomas of the hands and arms can occur in people who keep tropical fish in tanks. The cause may be an infection with *Mycobacterium marineum*, with which fish can be infected.

Fitz-Hugh–Curtis syndrome

Fitz-Hugh–Curtis syndrome is a perihepatic infection and fibrosis resulting from a gonococcal or chlamydial infection in women. Clinical features include fever, nausea, vomiting and upper right abdominal quadrant pain which can radiate into the back or right shoulder.

Focal dermal hypoplasia syndrome. See Goltz syndrome

Forbes–Albright syndrome

Forbes–Albright syndrome is galactorrhoea (excessive persistent lactation) due to an excessive production of prolactin by a pituitary tumour.

Foster–Kennedy syndrome

Other name Kennedy syndrome

Foster–Kennedy syndrome is characterized by optic atrophy and papilloedema on one side, sometimes with anosmia (absence of the sense of smell), due to a tumour on the under surface of a frontal lobe or a meningioma of the optic nerve.

Foville syndrome

Foville syndrome is a paralysis of the sixth and seventh cranial nerves, with hemiplegia on the opposite side. It is due to a lesion in the pons – usually an infarction or tumour – involving the fibres of the sixth and seventh cranial nerves fibres and motor fibres to the opposite side of the body. Other features can be Horner syndrome, loss of taste, deafness and analgesia on the affected side of the face.

Fragile X syndrome

Fragile X syndrome is a form of sex-linked mental retardation (IQ 30–60), which can be associated with large testes, slight enlargement of the head, prominent ears, laxity of joints, and fits. There is fragility of a particular site on a X chromosome, diagnosable by special cytogenetic studies. The frequency is about 0.9/1000 male births, which makes it one of the most common causes of mental retardation in boys. Female heterozygotes may be slightly mentally retarded.

Franceschetti–Jodassohn syndrome

Other name Naegli syndrome

Pigmentation of the skin beginning at 2 years of age on the arms and upper part of the trunk is associated with yellow teeth, hyperkeratosis of the palms and soles, excessive sweating and heat intolerance.

François syndrome. See Hallerman–Streiff syndrome

Freeman–Sheldon syndrome

Other names Whistling face; craniocarpotarsal dysplasia

Freeman–Sheldon syndrome is an autosomal dominant condition in which the central area of the face bulges as if the patient were whistling, probably due to a defect of the facial musculature. The face is stiff and mask-like. The mouth is small and pursed. Bilateral talipes equinovarus can be present. Intelligence and life span are probably normal.

Freiberg syndrome

Other names Freiberg infarction; osteochondrosis of a metatarsal head

Freiberg syndrome is an avascular necrosis of a metatarsal head, usually the second, and is characterized by localized pain and swelling over the metatarsal head and limitation of movement in an adolescent. X-rays show the head to be crushed and fragmented.

Frey syndrome

Other name Gustatory sweating

Frey syndrome is characterized by warmth and sweating in the malar region of the face on eating or thinking or talking about food. It may follow damage in the parotid region by trauma, mumps, purulent infection or surgery. It is thought that autonomic fibres to salivary glands have become connected in error with the sweat glands when they become reconnected after the damage which originally caused their connections to be interrupted. It can persist for life.

Froin syndrome

The cerebrospinal fluid, obtained by lumbar puncture, is yellow and the protein content is raised. It is an indication of a spinal block.

Frontal lobe syndrome

Other name Frontal lobishness

Damage to the frontal lobes causes changes in personality and behaviour. Common features are apathy, retardation, and an inability to plan activities, to carry them out and to anticipate the consequences of actions. There may be uncontrollable explosive attacks of rage, aggressive behaviour, bawdy talk and obstinacy. Damage to one lobe can cause hemiplegia on the opposite side and, if it is the dominant frontal lobe, there is likely also to be agraphia and a motor speech disorder. If both lobes are involved there can also be bilateral hemiplegia, spastic bulbar palsy and incontinence.

Fuchs syndromes

There are two syndromes. First, a progressive localized oedema of the eyelids. Secondly, a congenital progressive disorder of the eye, with heterochromia (a difference in colour between the irises or differences of colour in the same iris), uveitis of the lighter coloured eye, iridocyclitis (inflammation of the iris and ciliary body), keratitic precipitates and often cataract.

G

G syndrome. See Opitz–Frias syndrome

Gaillard syndrome

Gaillard syndrome is a displacement of the heart into the right side of the thorax due to collapse of the right lung or adhesions.

Ganser syndrome

Ganser syndrome is the giving of stupid answers to simple questions such as 10 when asked what 2 and 2 make. It can be a form of malingering or a hysterical response to stress.

Gardner syndrome

Gardner syndrome is an autosomal dominant inherited disorder characterized by polyposis coli, bone tumours, epidermoid cysts, desmoid tumours, odontomes (a solid cystic tumour of the jaw, derived from cells involved in tooth development) and unerupted teeth. Malignant changes develop in the intestinal polyps in about one third of cases.

Gardner–Diamond syndrome

Other names Painful bruising syndrome; autoerythrocyte sensitization syndrome; psychogenic purpura

Gardner–Diamond syndrome is a syndrome of uncertain origin occurring almost entirely in women. Precipitating factors are trauma, surgery and psychological disturbances and in part the lesions may be factitious (made by the patient). Clinical features are tingling, itching, pain and tenderness in the extremities, and painful nodules, which are red at first and later haemorrhagic. The prognosis is variable: in some patients the lesions persist for years, in others they clear up spontaneously within a few months. It was originally thought that the features were the result of extravasated blood causing the production of a skin-sensitizing antibody (hence the name of autoerythrocyte sensitization syndrome) but this has not been confirmed and there seems to be a strong psychological element in their production (hence the name of psychological purpura).

Gastrocutaneous syndrome

Gastrocutaneous syndrome is an autosomal dominant inherited syndrome characterized by peptic ulcer, hiatus hernia, myopia, hypertelorism (wide spacing of the eyes), multiple freckles and *café au lait* spots.

Gender dysphoria syndrome

The gender dysphoria syndrome is an emotional state characterized by restlessness, anxiety and depression in people who are unhappy with their sex and seek surgical alteration of their genital organs. They can be transsexuals, effeminate male homosexuals, transvestites, gross neurotics with impulses towards their genitalia, severe psychopaths or sociopaths, or psychotics with a delusion about their sexual identity.

General adaptation syndrome

General adaptation syndrome is the non-specific reactions produced by severe stress. It has been divided into Stage I of shock, Stage II of resistance and Stage III of exhaustion.

General neurotic syndrome

General neurotic syndrome is the concept that a patient may at various times in his life show features of various neuroses – such as anxiety, depressive illness, obsessive-compulsive states, phobias and panic disorders – formerly regarded as separate disorders, and that to react to stress in one of these ways is evidence of a personality factor predisposing to neurosis.

Genital retraction syndrome

Other name Koro

Genital retraction syndrome can occur after a stroke and principally in Chinese and Indonesian people. A male patient becomes deluded that his penis is shrinking, that it will disappear into his abdomen, and that this will kill him. A woman believes that her labia and breasts are shrinking with the same fatal result. It can occur as part of a severe anxiety or depression and can be regarded as part of a depersonalization syndrome.

German syndrome

Multiple fetal defects including mid-facial hypoplasia can be due to trimethadione or paramethadione taken by the mother during pregnancy.

Gerstmann syndrome

Disease of the association area of the dominant parietal lobe of the brain produces a disintegration of the patient's ability to recognize his body image. He mistakes the right and left sides of his body and cannot name his fingers. The ability to write and do sums may be affected.

Gerstmann–Strausler syndrome

Gerstmann–Strausler syndrome is a widespread degeneration of the nervous system, starting usually in the fourth decade of life and causing dementia. The cause is unknown: it is thought possible that it might be either a 'slow virus' or a prion (a particle of which little is known).

Gianotti–Crosti syndrome

Other name Infantile papular acrodermatitis

A non-itching erythematous papular eruption on the face and limbs is associated with enlarged lymph nodes and an enlarged liver. The eruption can become purpuric. There is an association with hepatitis B surface antigen. It is most common in Mediterranean countries.

Giant platelet syndrome. See Bernard–Soulier syndrome

Gilbert syndrome

Other name Familial unconjugated hyperbilirubinaemia

This inherited deficiency of the enzyme UDP glucuronyl transferase causes intermittent attacks of mild jaundice, abdominal pain or discomfort, weakness and fatigue. The liver is not enlarged. Urine is normal in colour. Bilirubin in unconjugated, and the results of transaminase determination are normal.

Gilles de la Tourette syndrome

Gilles de la Tourette syndrome is a disorder of unknown origin. It can be familial with an autosomal dominant inheritance. It begins in the first two decades of life and is likely to become chronic. The majority of cases are mild and undetected. It is characterized by multiple tics, grunts, coughs, sniffs, coprolalia (shouting out obscene words), echolalia (involuntarily repeating the words of others) and sometimes echopraxia (involuntarily repeating the actions of others). Associated features can be anxiety, obsessional-compulsive behaviour (with which it may be aetiologically and genetically related), sleep disturbances, stammering and self-injury.

Girdle syndrome

Girdle syndrome is pain in the lumbar region, clinical deterioration, a silent distended abdomen and respiratory failure, occurring as complications of sickle cell anaemia.

Gitlin syndrome

Gitlin syndrome is a mild form of Swiss-type agammaglobulinaemia with combined B-cell and T-cell deficiency, lymphopenia and recurrent respiratory and skin infections from the 2nd month of life.

Gjessing syndrome

Gjessing syndrome is a rare form of periodic stupor often with minor electroencephalographic (EEG) abnormalities during the stupor.

Glanzmann syndrome

Other name Thrombasthenia

In this familial syndrome there is a failure of platelets to aggregate. The platelets are normal in number. Clinical features are epistaxis, bruising and excessive bleeding after trauma.

Glanzmann–Riniker syndrome

Other name X-linked hypogammaglobulinaemia

Glanzmann–Riniker syndrome is an agammaglobulinaemia with aplasia of the thymus and aplasia of both T cells and B cells.

Glucagonoma syndrome

Other name Necrolytic migratory erythema

A migratory erythema of the trunk, limbs and the perioral and perigenital regions with blistering, desquamation and superficial skin necrosis can occur in patients with a glucagon-secreting pancreatic tumour.

Goldberg–Maxwell syndrome. See Testicular feminization syndrome

Goldenhar syndrome

Other name Oculo-auriculo-vertebral dysplasia

Goldenhar syndrome is characterized by multiple ocular, skeletal and other abnormalities: (a) coloboma of the upper eyelids and iris, subconjunctival lipoma, epibulbar dermoid, cataracts, glaucoma and strabismus; (b) fusion of vertebrae, elongation of the odontoid process of the mandible, cleft or highly-arched palate; (c) sensorineural deafness, renal abnormalities, congenital heart disease (commonly Fallot's tetralogy and septal defects) and mental retardation.

Goltz syndrome

Other name Focal dermal hypoplasia syndrome

Goltz syndrome is a multisystem disorder. Of reported cases, 88% have been female. It is thought that an X-linked dominant inheritance with lethality in the male is the likely form of inheritance.

Clinical features vary from mild to severe, and they vary too in the organs involved; cutaneous disorders have occurred in almost all cases. They are present at birth. They can be pink or red macules from a few millimetres to several centimetres across and sometimes blistered or eroded (a condition called cutis aplasia), telangiectasia, pinkish or brown nodules, as raspberry-like papillomas on the face, ears, fingers, toes and perianal region. The hair is sparse and brittle and there can be patches of alopecia. The nails can be dystrophic or absent. There can be skeletal deformities such as absence, hypoplasia or syndactyly of digits, lobster-claw deformity of the hands, scoliosis, and asymmetry in size and shape of the face, trunk and limbs. Longitudinal striations (osteopathia striata) are visible in the shafts of long bones on X-ray. Other deformities can be spina bifida, dysplasia of the clavicle, dental abnormalities, horseshoe kidney, exomphalos and other hernia, strabismus, low-set ears, microcephaly, development delay and recurrent infections. Intelligence is usually normal, but mental retardation has been reported in 15% of cases. Most patients can lead a normal life.

Goodpasture syndrome

Other names Haemorrhagic pulmonary-renal syndrome; pulmonary haemosiderosis with glomerulonephritis; lung purpura with nephritis; haemorrhagic and intestinal pneumonitis with nephritis

Goodpasture syndrome is characterized by glomerulonephritis and pulmonary haemorrhage. The aetiology is unknown. It can present at any age and is most common in young men. The glomerulonephritis is produced by antibodies against the glomerular membrane; it is shown by proteinuria and haematuria and is a cause of hypertension. Haemoptysis, which can vary from slight to massive, is the usual presenting feature. Haemorrhage into the alveoli causes impaired gas exchange and a decrease in pulmonary compliance, with the development of pulmonary fibrosis. Repeated haemoptyses produces anaemia. The prognosis is poor but some patients can survive for a long time and spontaneous remission has been reported. Death is usually due to a massive haemoptysis or renal or pulmonary failure.

Gorlin–Cohen syndrome

Other name Frontometaphyseal dysplasia

Gorlin–Cohen syndrome consists of facial asymmetry, mandibular hypoplasia, restrictive lung disease, primary pulmonary hypertension, bradycardia and skeletal abnormalities. Other features can be laryngomalacia (which can cause stridor), vocal cord paralysis and subglottic stenosis. The encephalogram (EEG) shows abnormalities. Intubation for an anaesthetic in an infant can be difficult.

Gradenigo syndrome

Gradenigo syndrome is characterized by pain in the face, due to irritation of the trigeminal nerve, and paralysis of the abducens nerve. It occurs most commonly as a complication of otitis media. Other causes are meningitis over the petrous part of the temporal bone or a tumour of the same region.

Graft-versus-host syndrome

Graft-versus-host syndrome is caused by foreign immunocompetent lymphoid cells encountering new antigens in a recipient capable of rejecting the cells. It is seen in patients with malignant disease who have received transplants of allogenic bone marrow and in patients with congenital immunodeficiencies given blood transfusions. The acute form appears within 100 days of transplantation, commonly 7–10 days after; clinical features are fever, diarrhoea and maculopapular rash on the trunk, palms, soles and oral mucous membrane. The chronic form appears after 100 days; clinical features are darkening and sclerosis of the skin and contractures; nails and hair may be shed.

Graham–Little syndrome

Graham–Little syndrome is a progressive cicatricial alopecia of the scalp and sometimes of the axillary and pubic regions, associated with keratosis pili (hyperkeratosis of the hair follicles), which is sometimes widespread.

Greig syndrome

Other name Ocular hypertelorism

Greig syndrome is an association of mental retardation with hypertelorism (wide spacing of the eyes) and other congenital lesions.

Grey syndrome

Maternal ingestion of chloramphenicol is said to have produced ashen grey cyanosis of the newborn baby, with cardiac arrest, cardiovascular collapse and respiratory failure. The fetal bone marrow may have been depressed.

Groenblad–Strandberg syndrome

Other name Pseudoxanthoma elasticum

Groenblad–Strandberg syndrome is a hereditary disorder of elastic tissue of which there are four genetically distinct variants. Degenerated elastic fibres are present in the skin, blood vessels and heart. Clinical features are soft yellowish papules in the skin, choroiditis and angioid streaks in the retina, bruising, haematemesis, angina pectoris and hypertension.

Guillain–Barré syndrome

Other names Landry–Guillain–Barré syndrome; acute idiopathic polyneuritis; acute infective polyneuritis

Guillain–Barré syndrome is the commonest form of acquired neuropathy. It is an acute mainly motor demyelinating polyneuropathy, which can appear 1 or 2 weeks after a febrile illness or after surgery. Clinical features are pain in the back and the legs and weakness beginning in the feet and legs and progressing upwards. The respiratory muscles are affected in about half the cases, and this puts the patient in danger. Involvement of the cranial nerves occurs sometimes. The tendon reflexes are lost. The condition is at its worst about 4 weeks after the onset. Spontaneous resolution is probably within 3–4 months, but can take up to 2 years. Some patients are left with some permanent weakness. Recurrence can occur in a few patients. The Fisher variant presents with facial weakness.

See also Acute relapsing Landry–Guillain–Barré syndrome

Gunn syndrome. See Marcus–Gunn syndrome

Haemangioma-thrombocytopenia syndrome. See Kasabach–Merritt syndrome

Haemoglobin Barts hydrops syndrome

When there is deletion of all four genes on chromosome 16 coding for the alpha globin chains, the only haemoglobin that can be synthesized in the second half of fetal life is Hb Barts (Y_4) which is not a good carrier of oxygen. The fetus is severely anaemic and oedematous and dies either late in pregnancy or shortly after birth. The mother has a high incidence of obstructed labour, postpartum haemorrhage and toxaemia.

Haemolytic-uraemic syndrome

Haemolytic-uraemic syndrome is characterized by acute renal failure, haemolytic anaemia and thrombocytopenia. It occurs mainly in infants; it can occur in adults, and in women there may be an association with pregnancy. It can follow an acute viral or bacterial infection and there is an association with *Salmonella* and *Shigella* infections. It can appear in a mild form, a severe acute form and a severe progressive form.

Prodromal symptoms, occurring a few days or weeks before the onset of the full syndrome, are diarrhoea, which may be bloody, vomiting and sometimes haematemesis. The full syndrome is characterized by abdominal pain, oliguria, petechiae, hypertension, congestive heart failure and convulsions; an acute abdominal condition can be mimicked. The blood shows thrombocytopenia, severe anaemia and abnormally shaped red cells. Renal disease can vary from a slight transitory functional decrease to a fulminant renal failure, which can go on to chronic renal failure. Involvement of the central nervous system is shown by irritability, fits, hemiparesis, drowsiness and coma. The liver and spleen can be enlarged and liver enzymes raised; jaundice is rare. Death can be due to renal failure or cerebral thrombosis.

Haemorrhagic pulmonary-renal syndrome. See Goodpasture syndrome

Hallermann-Streiff syndrome

Other names Dyscephalia mandibulo-oculofacialis; mandibulo-facial-dyscephaly; François syndrome

Hallermann-Streiff syndrome is a syndrome of multiple congenital abnormalities which can include malformations of the skull and facial bones, short stature, scoliosis, spina bifida, sensorineural deafness, beaked nose, hypoplastic nares, hypoplastic mandible, malocclusion of teeth, absent, extra or brittle teeth, diminished scalp and body hair, sparse or absent eyebrows and eyelashes, microphthalmia, cataracts, renal malformations, absence of radial bones and hypoplastic bone marrow.

Hallervorden–Spatz syndrome

Hallervorden–Spatz syndrome is an autosomal recessive inherited disorder in which there is a degeneration of the basal ganglia of the brain and the deposit of iron in them. The onset is in late childhood. Clinical features are athetosis, ataxia, rigidity, dysarthria, chorea and mental degeneration. The condition is progressive and causes death within a few years.

Hamman–Rich syndrome

Other names Fibrosing alveolitis; diffuse interstitial fibrosis of the lungs

Hamman–Rich syndrome is a progressive fibrosing alveolitis of the lungs in childhood, of unknown origin, consisting of respiratory embarrassment, cyanosis and right-sided heart failure. It is usually fatal.

Hand–foot syndrome

Hand–foot syndrome is characterized by pain, swelling and tenderness in either foot or hand due to micro-infarction of the carpal or tarsal bones with fever and leukocytosis. It occurs as a complication of sickle cell anaemia. It is self-limited, but there can be permanent radiological signs and it can recur. There is no permanent damage to the bones.

Hand–heart syndrome. See Holt–Oram syndrome

Hand–Schüller–Christian syndrome

Other names Histiocytosis X; Letterer–Siwe disease

Hand–Schüller–Christian syndrome is a group of disorders characterized by histiocytic granulomas in various tissues. The usual site is the skull; other sites are the lungs, liver, lymph nodes and skin. Clinical features include evidence of the bony lesions, diabetes insipidus, otitis externa, skin rashes, gingivitis, lipoidosis and fibrosis of the lungs. In Letterer–Siwe disease the lesions are widespread, the disease is severe and death likely within a short time.

Happy puppet syndrome

In happy puppet syndrome severe mental retardation is associated with jerky movements as if the child were being jerked by strings like a puppet, an open-mouth expression, outbursts of laughter and poor physical development.

Harada syndrome

Harada syndrome is Vogt–Koyanagi syndrome plus retinal detachment due to exudative choroiditis.

Harlequin syndrome

Harlequin syndrome is characterized by sudden unilateral flushing and sweating developing spontaneously or in response to heat, exercise or eating spicy food.

Hartnup syndrome

This autosomal recessive disorder of amino acid metabolism is characterized by mental retardation, episodes of cerebellar ataxia and a photosensitive rash. It is named after the patient in whom it was first diagnosed.

Hartnup-like syndrome

In this disorder of tryptophan metabolism an increased amount of tryptophan remains with the intestinal contents, and there is an increased production of tryptophan by intestinal micro-organisms, with the production of a condition resembling Hartnup syndrome.

Heerfordt syndrome

Other name Uveoparotid fever

Heerfordt syndrome is a form of sarcoidosis with enlargement of the parotid glands, fever and uveitis.

HELLP syndrome

HELLP syndrome is:

H – haemolysis
EL – elevated liver enzymes
LP – low platelet count.

The syndrome occurs in severe pre-eclampsia with progressive liver function deterioration in a pregnant woman and is arrestable only by delivery.

Hemichorea–hemiballismus syndrome

Hemichorea–hemiballismus syndrome is one of the 'lacunar syndromes' in which small spaces are present in the brain. In this syndrome they appear in the subthalamic regions with sparing of the internal capsule and cause hemichorea (choreic movements of one side of the body) and hemiballismus (violent flinging movements of one side of the body).

Henoch–Schönlein syndrome

Other names Anaphylactoid purpura; allergic purpura; purpura rheumatica

Henoch–Schönlein syndrome is an allergic reaction to bacteria (especially β-haemolytic streptococci), food or drugs. It usually presents 1–3 weeks after an upper respiratory tract infection. It can occur at any age but it is most common in childhood and adolescence with the age of onset usually between 6 months and 6 years. It accounts for up to 15% of cases of glomerular nephropathy in children. Clinical features are a purpuric, maculopapular or urticarial rash on the extensor surfaces of the arms and legs, nephritis (beginning about 4 weeks after the onset of the illness), swelling and tenderness of joints and a localized painful oedema of the scalp, feet and hands. Gastrointestinal bleeding can cause colicky abdominal pain, haematemesis and melaena. Intussusception can follow oedema of the bowel or haemorrhage into it. Subcutaneous bleeding can occur in the eyelids, conjunctiva, calves (mimicking a deep-vein thrombosis), and scrotum (mimicking torsion of the testis). Other features can be nose-bleeds, an enlarged liver, intracranial oedema and haemorrhage, oedema of the epiglottis and, rarely, chorea, fits, facial palsy and encephalopathy. The white cell count and erythrocyte sedimentation rate are raised. The neuropathy can progress to renal failure.

Hepatic encephalopathy syndrome

Progressive liver failure produces an encephalopathy characterized by impaired consciousness, impaired mental functions, personality changes, tremor, focal or general fits, delirium, stupor and coma.

Hepatorenal syndrome

Other name Hepatonephric syndrome

Hepatorenal syndrome is acute renal failure occurring in a patient with cirrhosis of the liver or disease of the biliary tract.

Her syndrome

Other name Hepatic phosphorylase deficiency

Her syndrome is a glycogen storage disorder with deficiency of hepatic phosphorylase associated with an enlarged liver and mild hypoglycaemia.

Hermansky–Pudlak syndrome

Other name Hermansky syndrome

Hermansky–Pudlak syndrome is a hereditary platelet defect causing haem-orrhages associated with albinism and accumulation of a ceroid-like material in the lungs, oral mucosa, intestinal mucosa and reticulo-endothelial system. Characteristic features are bruising, haemoptysis, epistaxis, gingival bleeding, bleeding after tooth extraction, loss of pigment from the skin, hair and irises and intestinal pulmonary fibrosis. Renal failure, cardiac failure and ulcerative colitis can occur.

HHE syndrome

HHE syndrome is:

    H – hemiplegia
    H – hemiconvulsions
    E – epilepsy.

HHE syndrome is the occurrence of hemiplegia, convulsions involving one side of the body and other epileptic seizures occurring in childhood, usually as a complication of an acute febrile illness.

High T$_4$ syndrome. See Euthyroid sick syndrome

Hinman syndrome

Other name Dysfunctional voiding

Hinman syndrome is an association in childhood of enuresis, frequency and urge incontinence by day, which can be complicated by urinary tract infection and renal damage, which can progress to end-stage renal disease.

Hippel–Lindau syndrome

Other name Lindau–Hippel syndrome

Hippel–Lindau syndrome is an autosomal dominant condition characterized by angiomatous tumours of the retina, cutaneous naevi, haemangioblastoma of the cerebellum and spinal cord, a cerebellar syndrome, increased intracranial pressure, angiomatous or cystic lesions of the liver, pancreas, kidneys, lungs, epididymis and skin, phaeochromocytoma and renal cell carcinoma. The retinal angiomas can cause haemorrhages into the eye, retinal detachment and blindness. Hepatic and renal failure can occur. Neurofibromatosis (Recklinghausen's disease) can be an associated condition. The prognosis is poor and death is likely to occur from these failures, an intracranial haemorrhage or a cerebellar tumour.

Hoffmann–Zurhelle syndrome

Other name Naevus lipomatides superficialis

Hoffmann–Zurhelle syndrome is a developmental abnormality of the skin in which soft fleshy nodules, usually present at birth, are found in the skin, especially on the lower part of the trunk.

Hoigne syndrome. See Stress response syndrome

Holmes–Adie syndrome

Other names Adie syndrome; tonic pupil

One pupil is dilated and reacts very slowly to light and a near stimulus. If the patient is in a darkened room for some time a bright light can cause slow and incomplete constriction of the pupil. The pupil usually constricts in response to drops of methacholine 5%, indicating a supersensitivity to acetylcholine. The patient may complain of sensitivity to light in the affected eye. The lesion is in the ciliary ganglion.

It is most common in women aged 20–40 years. Orbital surgery and viral infection can be causes, but in most cases the cause is unknown. If the condition develops suddenly the patient may complain of subjective visual disturbance due to the loss of accommodation. The knee and ankle jerks are usually absent. Other associated conditions are cardiac dysrhythmias and Ross syndrome (segmental loss of sweating).

Holiday heart syndrome

Holiday heart syndrome is any cardiac arrhythmia provoked by an alcoholic binge as can occur at a weekend or during a holiday.

Holt–Oram syndrome

Other name Hand–heart syndrome

In this autosomal dominant disorder congenital cardiovascular malformations (commonly an atrial septal defect) are associated with an upper limb defect (usually of the radius or thumb) in one person or separately in different members of a family. It is divided into two types: the complete type has both cardiovascular and upper limb deformities; the incomplete type has either the cardiovascular or the upper limb deformities.

Hopkins–Neville–Bannister syndrome

Hopkins–Neville–Bannister syndrome is an acute autonomic neuropathy characterized by diarrhoea, ileus, postural hypotension and bladder dysfunction, especially urinary retention.

Horner syndrome

Horner syndrome is characterized by ptosis, miosis (small pupil), enophthalmos (sinking back of the eyeball into the orbit), diminished or absent facial sweating – all on one side. It can be congenital or be due to an injury of the cervical sympathetic chain or its involvement in a tumour or vascular accident. If it occurs early in childhood, pigmentation of the iris on that side may be delayed or different from that on the other side. It occurs in about half the patients who have had interscalene or subclavian perivascular anaesthetic blocks.

Houssay syndrome

In a patient with diabetes mellitus an infarction of the pituitary gland or surgical removal of the gland can produce hypoglycaemia.

Howel–Evans syndrome

A diffuse hypertrophy of the horny layer of the skin of the palms and sole appears between the ages of 5 and 15 years and is frequently associated with carcinoma of the oesophagus.

Hughes–Stovin syndrome

Hughes–Stovin syndrome is an association of segmental pulmonary artery aneurysms with peripheral venous thrombosis. Clinical features are recurrent thromboses of superficial and deep veins, haemoptysis, progressive dyspnoea and cyanosis, and often signs of pulmonary hypertension. Death can be due to rupture of a pulmonary aneurysm.

Hunter syndrome

Other name Mucopolysaccharidosis type II

In this sex-linked recessive disorder there is a deficiency of iduronate acid sulphatase and an abnormal deposit of mucopolysaccharides in various tissues. An affected child may appear normal up to about 1 year of life. Clinical features include short stature, coarse facies, an enlarged liver and spleen, stiff joints, thoracoskeletal deformities which can cause respiratory failure, laryngeal and pharyngeal obstruction, cardiac infiltration and failure, mental retardation and behaviour problems. Other features can be ivory-coloured nodules in the skin, progressive loss of sight and hearing, hydrocephalus and a degeneration of central nervous system functioning. It is usually less severe than Hurler syndrome. Many patients die in childhood, but those with a minor form of the disorder can survive to early adult life.

It can be diagnosed *in utero* by an assay of iduronate acid sulphatase in fetal blood.

Hurler syndrome

Other name Mucopolysaccharidosis type I

Hurler syndrome is an autosomal recessive inherited mucopolysaccharidosis in which there is a deficiency of α-L-iduronidase and an abnormal deposit of mucopolysaccharides in many tissues, especially noticeable in the brain, cornea, liver, spleen and bone. An affected child may appear normal up to about 1 year of life and then the head may be noticed to be becoming abnormally large. Clinical features are likely to include a large and abnormally shaped head, a short thick neck, growth retardation, coarse facies, large tongue, hyperplastic gums, abnormally shaped and widely spaced teeth, corneal opacities, glaucoma, sensorineural deafness, an enlarged liver and spleen, a protuberant abdomen, umbilical and inguinal hernias, coronary artery thickening, angina pectoris, myocardial infarction, decreased joint mobility and frequent chest infections. X-rays show bony abnormalities, including small wedge-shaped vertebrae. Death usually occurs before 10 years of age.

It can be diagnosed *in utero* by assay of α-L-iduronidase in the fetal blood.

Hutchinson–Gilford syndrome

Other name Progeria

Hutchinson–Gilford syndrome is a very rare disease of young children; it is possibly inherited as an autosomal recessive disorder. The affected child has a very old appearance, which can be partly present at birth or develops within the first 10 years of life. The face is prematurely wrinkled with small jaws, often protruding eyes, enlarged scalp veins and sparse growth of hair. Later features are premature greying of the hair and alopecia, growth stagnation and arteriosclerosis. Intelligence is usually normal. Affected children usually die before the age of 20 years from the effects of arteriosclerosis.

Hypereosinophilic syndrome

This multiple-system disorder is most common in middle-aged men and is of unknown aetiology. There is an excess of eosinophils (in the absence of any known cause of eosinophilia) and damage is caused by the excess of hydrolytic enzymes and major basic protein released from the eosinophils. Clinical features can include fever, malaise, weight loss, abdominal pain, cough, joint pain, enlarged liver, enlarged spleen, endocardial fibrosis, restrictive endomyocarditis, mitral regurgitation, tricuspid regurgitation, congestive heart failure, papular or urticarial rashes, dermographism, polyneuropathy and mental disturbances. With treatment about 80% have a 5-year survival. Death is usually due to heart failure, renal failure, liver failure, haemorrhage or infection.

Hyperimmunoglobin E recurrent infection syndrome. See Job syndrome

Hyperkinetic heart syndrome

Hyperkinetic heart syndrome is most likely to occur in males between the ages of 10 and 50 years. Clinical features are palpitations, a pounding sensation in the chest, pounding peripheral pulses, ejection-type systolic murmurs, systolic ejection clicks and, sometimes, left ventricular hypertrophy. Haemodynamic findings are a high cardiac output and increased ejection rate per beat. The electrocardiograph will show evidence of left ventricular hypertrophy if it is present.

Hyperkinetic syndrome

This mental disorder of childhood (most commonly in mentally retarded, epileptic or brain-damaged children) is characterized by overactivity, disruptive behaviour, impairment of attention and impairment of learning.

Hyperventilation syndrome

Hyperventilation syndrome is characterized by attacks of hyperventilation usually occurring when the patient is at rest. The over-breathing causes hypocapnoea, which in turn causes cerebral vasoconstriction, alkalosis and a shift of the haemoglobin oxygen dissociation curve with a reduction of the supply of oxygen to the tissues, and in particular to the central nervous system. The condition is most common in women, and stress is often a factor in the production of attacks. The attack of rapid deep breathing can be followed by giddiness, paraesthesia (sometimes one-sided), blurred vision, headache, ataxia, tremulousness and loss of consciousness. The patient may be thought to have epilepsy. Other symptoms can be nausea, vomiting and palpitations. Between attacks the patient may complain of headache, insomnia, tiredness, motor weakness, chest discomfort and abdominal discomfort. The acute symptoms can be relieved by the patient rebreathing into a paper bag held over the nose and mouth.

Hyperviscosity syndrome

The plasma viscosity can be raised in 'high cell states', e.g. leukaemia, and 'high protein states', e.g. myeloma, Waldenström's macroglobulinaemia. The cerebral blood flow is reduced. Clinical features include headache, dizziness, drowsiness, transient ischaemic attacks, aphasia and the effects of thrombotic episodes. Papilloedema and blurring or loss of vision can occur as the result of blood stasis in the retina and occlusion of the central retinal vein.

Hypoplastic left heart syndrome

Hypoplastic left heart syndrome can be due to a number of congenital abnormalities of the left side of the heart and great vessels. The abnormalities include hypoplasia of the left ventricle, hypoplasia of the ascending aorta (which supplies only the coronary arteries), mitral atresia or stenosis, aortic atresia or stenosis, and coarctation of the aorta where the ductus arteriosus enters it. The ductus arteriosus is large and remains patent, and the body (except for the heart) is supplied with the blood that passes through it.

Hypoplastic right heart syndrome

Hypoplastic right heart syndrome is due to a number of congenital abnormalities of the right side of the heart. These abnormalities can include hypoplasia of the right ventricle, hypoplasia or stenosis of the pulmonary artery, atresia of the tricuspid valve and atresia or stenosis of the pulmonary valve.

Hypospadias-dysphagia syndrome. See Opitz–Frias syndrome

I

IBIDS syndrome

IBIDS syndrome is an autosomal recessive disorder characterized by:

I – ichthyosis
B – brittle hair
I – impairment, physical and mental
D – decreased fertility
S – short stature.

See also BIDS syndrome

Idiopathic long Q-T syndrome

A prolonged Q-T interval on an electrocardiogram (EEG) is thought to be due to an imbalance between right and left sympathetic activity. Low right-sided sympathetic activity results in left-sided dominance and an increase in ventricular dispersion or repolarization. Many cases are sporadic with no family history but some may have an autosomal recessive transmission with or without congenital deafness. Associated features can be sinus bradycardia, a slow pulse rate and abnormal T waves, which can be bifid, biphasic or notched. Patients may have syncopal attacks due to emotional, auditory or physical stimulation, and ventricular tachyarrhythmias can be triggered by emotional or physical stress. Sudden death is common.

See also Jervell–Lange-Nielsen syndrome; Romano–Ward syndrome

Idiopathic genetic syndromes

This term is used to describe the large numbers of genetic diseases which are variable in their clinical features, rare, overlapping in their clinical features and difficult to diagnose precisely.

Immature lung syndrome

Other name Primary atelectasis

Immature lung syndrome can occur in premature babies. The onset is about

8 hours after birth. Breathing is impaired by slow expansion of the lobes or recurrent collapse, chiefly of the lower lobes. Associated conditions can be congenital diaphragmatic hernia and a hypoplastic pulmonary artery.

Imerslund syndrome

Other name Imerslund–Graesbeck syndrome

In this type of megaloblastic anaemia there is a selective ileal malabsorption of vitamin B_{12} and proteinuria.

Immotile cilia syndrome

Other names Ciliary dyskinesia; Kartagener syndrome; Afzelius syndrome

Immotile cilia syndrome is an autosomal recessive inherited disorder in which there is an absence of the dyenin arms of cilia, arms which are essential for the mobility of the cilia, dyenin being a substance that can convert chemical energy into tubular contractility. Principal effects are on (a) the ciliated cells of the respiratory system, with a liability to develop bronchitis and bronchiectasis, and (b) spermatozoa, whose tails are affected and movements limited, with the production of infertility in male patients. Situs inversus (lateral transposition of the thoracic and abdominal viscera) or dextrocardia can be present. The mobility of polymorphonuclear leukocytes is defective. Other clinical features can be chronic otitis media, sinusitis and recurrent infections, with *Pneumococcus* and *Haemophilus* as the common infecting organisms.

Inappropriate antidiuretic hormone (ADH) secretion syndrome

Excessive production of ADH can be due to (a) endocrine disease: hypoadrenalism, hypopituitarism, hypothyroidism; (b) pulmonary disease: carcinoma of lung, pneumonia, bronchopneumonia, pulmonary tuberculosis, aspergillosis; (c) brain disease: cerebral tumour, cerebral abscess, cerebral haemorrhage, subarachnoid haemorrhage, subdural haemorrhage, cerebral thrombosis, head injury; (d) Guillain–Barré syndrome, acute intermittent porphyria, cirrhosis of the liver, various tumours, some drugs. It can occur postoperatively and idiopathically. The tubular reabsorption of water in the kidney is promoted and leads to severe hyponatraemia and hypo-osmolarity. The hyponatraemia can cause seizures and coma.

Inferior vena cava syndrome

Inferior vena cava syndrome is characterized by oedema of the legs and distension of superficial veins. It can be due to thrombosis of the inferior vena cava, invasion of the inferior vena cava by renal cell carcinoma, or pressure on the inferior vena cava by an aneurysm of the abdominal aorta. The nephrotic syndrome can be produced if the renal veins are involved and the Budd–Chiari syndrome if the hepatic veins are involved.

Inspissated bile syndrome

Inspissated bile syndrome is a severe jaundice, persisting for up to 2 months, with conversion of an indirect to a direct hyperbilirubinaemia following a severe haemolytic disease. It was attributed to plugs of thick bile obstructing the bile ducts, but pathological specimens show necrosis of liver cells, portal fibrosis and inflammatory changes similar to those of neonatal hepatitis.

Irritable bowel syndrome

Other names Mucous colitis; spastic colon

Irritable bowel syndrome is a motor disorder characterized by irregular bowel function with spells of both diarrhoea and constipation, the passing of much mucus and intermittent mild abdominal pain. Stress and deficiency of dietary fibre are factors in its production. About 70% of patients, especially women, have suffered from depression and may have considered suicide.

Irvine–Gass syndrome

Irvine–Gass syndrome is cystic macular oedema of the eye which occurs in about 50% of cases subjected to fluorescein angiography a few weeks after intrascapular extraction of a cataract. The oedema usually resolves over several months and there are no permanent ill effects. It occurs in less than 5% of extrascapular cataract extractions.

Isolation syndrome

Isolation syndrome can occur in old people in residential homes and without visitors or conversation with anyone. They become unable to make social contacts or to ask for help and sink into 'dumb' postures; their facial expressions and physical movements become frozen.

Ivemark syndrome. See Asplenia syndrome

J

Jackson syndrome

A softening or tumour of the tegmentum of the medulla oblongata causes Avellis syndrome plus paralysis of the tongue on the same side as the lesion.

Jacob syndrome

Conjunctivitis, stomatitis and scrotal dermatitis are due to a deficiency of riboflavin (vitamin B_2).

Jadassohn–Lewandowsky syndrome

Other name Pachyonychia congenita

Jadassohn–Lewandowsky syndrome is an autosomal dominant ectodermal dysplasia characterized by oral leukoplakia, dysplastic teeth present at birth, palmar and plantar keratosis (thickening of the horny layer of the skin), follicular keratosis of the elbows and knees, dystrophy of the nails and excessive perspiration.

Janz syndrome

Other name Myoclonic epilepsy of adolescence

Janz syndrome is characterized by myoclonus occurring bilaterally and especially in the upper limbs in adolescence, often after awakening. In girls it may be associated with menstruation. The patient may have major and minor epileptic seizures.

Jaw-winking syndrome. See Marcus–Gunn syndrome

Jervell–Lange-Nielsen syndrome

Other name Surdocardiac syndrome; cardio-auditory syndrome

Jervell–Lange-Nielsen syndrome is an autosomal recessive disorder characterized by congenital deaf-mutism and a long Q-T interval on an electrocardiogram. The aetiology is unknown. The long Q-T interval is thought to be due to a congenital anomaly of myocardial metabolism, with delay of the repolarization phase due to some enzyme deficiency. No gross abnormality of the heart is present. Paroxysmal ventricular fibrillation or tachycardia and fainting fits can occur. Sudden death in early childhood is likely.

See also Idiopathic long Q-T syndrome

Jessner–Kanof syndrome

Jessner–Kanof syndrome is a lymphocytic infiltration of the skin occurring mainly on the face. Small reddish papules appear and gradually enlarge peripherally, sometimes leaving the centre clear. They resolve spontaneously without leaving scars.

Jeune syndrome

Other name Asphyxiating thoracic dysplasia

Jeune syndrome is a familial disorder involving many bones. Deformities of the chest wall can contribute to asphyxial attacks which can be fatal.

Job syndrome

Other name Hyperimmunoglobin E recurrent infection syndrome

Job syndrome is an immunological disorder of unknown aetiology, affecting both males and females, in which there is overproduction of IgE and monocyte or neutrophil chemotactic deficiency. Clinical features are recurrent infections of the skin, sinuses and pulmonary tract, beginning in childhood. Infecting organisms are likely to be *Staphylococcus aureus*, *Pneumocystis carinii* and *Cryptococcus*. The characteristic feature is the presence of large abscesses, which contain a great deal of purulent material but with little inflammatory reaction. Other features can be a coarse facies, a chronic eczemoid rash, mucocutaneous candidiasis, nasal discharge, otitis media, fever and leukocytosis; red hair is common.

It is named after Job of the Bible who had multiple boils.

Josephs–Diamond–Blackfan syndrome

Other names Blackfan–Diamond syndrome; pure red cell aplasia; erythrogenesis imperfecta; congenital hypoplastic anaemia

This defect of red cell production becomes apparent at 3–12 months of age. The bone marrow shows a great reduction or almost complete absence of red cell precursors, and in consequence a severe anaemia is produced. There may be a slight neutropenia (diminished number of neutrophils in the blood) and thrombocytopenia (diminished number of platelets in the blood). The liver and spleen may become enlarged but these enlargements may be due to haemosiderosis (increase of iron in the tissues) following multiple blood transfusions.

Joubert syndrome

Joubert syndrome is characterized by episodic panting in the newborn and jerky eye movements in the neonatal period with later the development of mental retardation, ataxia and disequilibrium. Pathological features are brainstem malformation and agenesis of the vermis of the cerebellum.

Jugular foramen syndrome

Other name Vernet syndrome

In jugular foramen syndrome paralysis of the ninth, tenth and eleventh cranial nerves causes hoarseness, dysphagia and nasal regurgitation. The causes can be glomus jugulare tumour or, less commonly, trauma or a meningeal infiltration by tumour tissue involving the affected cranial nerves.

K

Kallmann syndrome

Kallmann syndrome is an association of hypogonadism, eunuchoidism and absence or poor sense of smell (due to degeneration of the olfactory bulbs). Midline cranial and intracranial defects and retinitis pigmentosa can be present. It is an inherited condition: X-linked and autosomal dominant and recessive modes of inheritance have all been reported.

Kanner syndrome

Other name Autism

Kanner syndrome is a serious disorder of early childhood usually presenting in the 2nd or 3rd years of life. The principal clinical features are: (a) detachment from the parents or others, who are treated as though they are not there, with avoidance of eye contact and a failure to develop normal social responses; (b) absence or abnormality of language development and speech, words learned may be lost, questions are not answered, intonation is abnormal; (c) behaviour abnormality, with temper tantrums, repetitive activities such as scribbling on a piece of paper or rubbing a toy up and down on the floor, walking on tiptoe, rocking, spinning round and round, grimacing; (d) obsessive interest in small things, patterns, music, puzzles. Many of the children are mentally retarded. The cause is unknown, but there is some evidence that there may be temporal lobe lesions and dysfunction. The prognosis is poor. Children of low intelligence do not recover and are likely to require care for life. Others may exist as detached loners with poor social relations, speech difficulties and behavioural abnormalities.

Kartagener syndrome. See Immotile cilia syndrome

Kasabach–Merritt syndrome

Other name Haemangioma-thrombocytopenia syndrome

In Kasabach–Merritt syndrome of infancy, a congenital haemangioma is associated with intravascular coagulation. The haemangioma can be small at first and rapidly growing or it can be large from the first; it is usually on a limb but it can be on the trunk or a viscus. Other features are purpura, thrombocytopenia, hypofibrinogenaemia and an increased amount of fibrinopeptide (a degradation product of fibrinogen). The clinical features can be mild and chronic, and the haemangioma, like other congenital haemangiomas, may resolve in time.

Kast syndrome. See Maffucci syndrome

Katayama syndrome

Fever, malaise, cough, urticaria, diarrhoea and an increase in the number of eosinophils can occur in the early stages of infection by *Schistosoma japonicum* or *Schistosoma mansoni*.

It is named after part of the island of Honshu, Japan.

Kawasaki syndrome

Kawasaki syndrome was first described by Kawasaki in Japanese children and since then it has been recognized in Europe and North America. The cause is uncertain. It can occur in small epidemics. The characteristic features are fever, a strawberry tongue, reddening of the oropharyngeal mucosa, conjunctivitis, a bright red erythema of the hands and feet, which become swollen and indurated, and a morbilliform maculopapular rash on the trunk and limbs within 5 days of the onset of the fever. Enlarged cervical lymph nodes occur in half to three-quarters of the patients. Indurative oedema and pain in the extremities are sometimes the predominant physical features. In the acute phase the coronary arteries can become dilated; this can lead to the development of aneurysms of the coronary arteries, and to death.

Kearns–Sayre syndrome

Other name Ophthalmoplegia plus

Kearns–Sayre syndrome is an abnormality of mitochondrial enzymes which causes a progressive ophthalmoplegia, cerebellar ataxia, and an increase in cerebrospinal fluid protein. Other features can be slight muscular weakness, retinal degeneration, sensory deafness, cardiomyopathy, myocardial conduction block, and short stature.

Kennedy syndrome. See Foster–Kennedy syndrome

Kienbock syndrome

Kienbock syndrome is an aseptic necrosis of the lunate bone due to ischaemia or inflammation.

Kimmelstiel–Wilson syndrome

Other name Glomerular hyalinization

Hyalinization of the renal glomeruli is a severe complication of diabetes mellitus. Proteinuria occurs. It begins about 15 years after the onset of diabetes and is commonly associated with retinopathy.

Kleine–Levin syndrome

Kleine–Levin syndrome is a disorder of unknown causation in young adult males and is characterized by long periods of hypersomnia and increased appetite and libido on wakening.

Klinefelter syndrome

Other name XXY syndrome

In Klinefelter syndrome an additional X chromosome (XXY karyotype) is associated with primary testicular failure. Common features are tall stature, slim build, poor sexual development, small hard testes, gynaecomastia (enlargement of the male breast) and infertility. Some patients can be below average intelligence. Crush fractures of osteoporotic vertebrae can occur. Subtypes can occur in which fertility is present.

Klippel–Feil syndrome

Klippel–Feil syndrome is a reduction in the number of cervical vertebrae or the fusion of multiple hemivertebrae into one causing shortness or stiffness of the neck and a low hair line.

Klippel–Trenaunay–Weber syndrome

Other names Klippel–Trenaunay syndrome; osteohypertrophic angioectases

Klippel–Trenaunay–Weber syndrome is characterized by multiple malformations of soft tissue and bone, including arteriovenous aneurysms, cutaneous telangiectasia, vascular hamartomas, syndactylism, polydactylism and cleft palate. Hypertrophy of bones and soft tissues occurs as a result of the increased flow of blood in the limbs. An arteriovenous shunt can lead to the development of high-output cardiac failure. The patient can have a short wide neck and may be unable to extend it; this can be an anaesthetic problem.

Kluver–Bucy syndrome

Kluver–Bucy syndrome is due to bilateral damage of the temporal lobes. It can occur in Alzheimer's disease, Pick's disease of the brain, Huntington's disease, trauma, vascular lesions, encephalitis, hypoglycaemia, toxoplasmosis, acute intermittent porphyria and adrenoleukodystrophy. Clinical features include severe loss of memory, abnormal sexual activities, emotional blunting, manual exploratory behaviour and attacks of 'sham rage'.

Köhler syndrome

Other name Osteochondritis of the tarsal navicular bone

Köhler syndrome is an avascular necrosis of the tarsal navicular bone, possibly due to repetitive compressive forces which cause a loss of blood supply and fragmentation in a bone that is not fully ossified. It occurs at the age of 4–5 years. The patient complains of pain over the bone and swelling over it is noticeable. X-ray shows either a collapse of the bone or increased density and fragmentation without a change in shape or size. It is usually a self-limited disorder which resolves with full ossification of the bone about 2 years later.

Korsakoff syndrome

Other name Korsakov syndrome

Korsakoff syndrome is characterized by a severe memory defect, especially for recent events, for which the patient compensates by confabulation (the reciting of imaginary experiences). It is a feature of chronic alcoholism and is due either to the direct effects of alcohol or to the severe nutritional deficiencies which are associated with chronic alcoholism.

Kostmann syndrome

Other name Congenital agranulocytosis

Kostmann syndrome is a congenital disorder characterized by severe neutropenia and maturation arrest at the myelocyte level. It runs a progressively downhill course with death usually within the 1st year of life and usually from *Pseudomonas* or *Staphylococcus aureus* pulmonary infection.

Krabbe syndrome

Other name Globoid cell leukodystrophy

In Krabbe syndrome there is a primary deficiency of the enzyme galactocerebrosidase. This causes demyelination and the presence of inclusion bodies in the Schwann cells. Spastic paralysis develops in infancy and progresses to a flaccid paralysis and death.

Kufs syndrome

In this adult-onset storage disorder there is an abnormal storage in the brain of lipofuscin, granular material and membrane fragments. Clinical features are spasticity, ataxia, myoclonus, fits, visual failure and dementia.

Kugelberg–Welander syndrome

Other name Wohlfahrt–Kugelberg–Welander syndrome

Kugelberg–Welander syndrome is a juvenile form of spinal muscular atrophy with limb and girdle weakness beginning in childhood and due to degeneration of anterior horn cells. Fasciculation (involuntary muscle contractions, due to discharge in a single motor nerve filament) and fibrillation (muscular contractions due to spontaneous activation of a single muscle cell or fibre) occur.

L

Laband syndrome

This autosomal dominant inherited disease is characterized by fibrosis of the gums, abnormalities of the ears, nose, nails and tips of the fingers and sometimes an enlarged liver and enlarged spleen.

Lactase deficiency syndrome

Deficiency of the disaccharide-splitting enzyme lactase can cause diarrhoea when a lactose-containing food such as milk is ingested.

Lacunar syndromes

These are a number of syndromes in which there are small cavities (originally called 'un état lacunaire') present in the cerebral substance. It is thought that they are the result of infarctions following the occlusion of arterioles, and they occur in middle-aged or elderly patients with atherosclerosis and hypertension. Multiple infarcts can cause difficulty in walking, pseudobulbar palsy and a progressive dementia.

LAMB syndrome

LAMB syndrome is characterized by:

 L – lentigenes (freckles)
 A – atrial myxoma
 M – mucous myxomas
 B – blue naevi.

It may be the same as NAME syndrome.

Lambert–Eaton syndrome

Other names Carcinomatous myasthenia; carcinomatous myopathy

Lambert–Eaton syndrome is a progressive muscular weakness in a patient with a carcinoma.

Landau–Kleffner syndrome

Other name Acquired epileptic aphasia

Landau–Kleffner syndrome is a disorder of childhood characterized by acquired aphasia, epileptic seizures, multiple focal epileptic spikes on an electroencephalogram (EEG), and behavioural and psychomotor disturbances.

Landry–Guillain–Barré syndrome. See Guillain–Barré syndrome

Langer–Gideon syndrome

Langer–Gideon syndrome is one of the contiguous gene syndromes. There is a combination of mental retardation and physical abnormalities. There is a deletion of part of chromosome 8, which is detectable by gene mapping or the use of restriction fragment length polymorphs.

Large atypical mole syndrome. See Familial atypical multiple mole-melanoma syndrome

Laron-type dwarfism phenotypic syndrome

Severe growth retardation with Laron phenotype is associated with chronic elevation of plasma growth hormone (GH) levels, resistance to the effects of exogenous growth hormone on growth and the generation of insulin-like growth factor I (IGF-1) and absence of the principal growth hormone-binding proteins.

Larsen syndrome

This familial disorder is characterized by a flat face, hypertelorism (wide spacing of the eyes) and a liability to multiple dislocations of joints. The soft palate can be cleft.

Larsen–Johansson syndrome

Other name Adolescent patellar chondromalacia

This is an inflammation of the lower accessory centre of ossification in the patella.

Laubenthal syndrome

Other name Xerodermic idiocy and ataxia

This congenital disorder is characterized by severe mental retardation, short stature, cerebellar ataxia, tremor and delayed dentition.

Laurence–Moon–Biedl syndrome

Other names Laurence–Biedl syndrome; Laurence–Moon–Bardet–Biedl syndrome

This autosomal recessive inherited condition is characterized by obesity, gonadal hypoplasia and retinitis pigmentosa. Associated conditions are spastic paraplegia, congenital heart defects, polydactylism, syndactylism, skull defects, diabetes mellitus and mental retardation.

Lawrence–Seip syndrome

Other name Lipoatrophy

This is a familial disorder of gigantism with loss of subcutaneous fat, hirsutism, diabetes mellitus and the late development of renal failure.

Lazy leukocyte syndrome

In lazy leukocyte syndrome leukocytes appear normal in the bone marrow but their locomotive ability is reduced, which reduces their ability to migrate from bone marrow into the circulation. This produces neutropenia. In the circulation the leukocytes' ability to move to sites of inflammation is reduced. The patient is likely to have frequent respiratory tract infections and stomatitis. A similar but transient syndrome is called 'transient lazy leukocyte syndrome'.

Leiner syndrome

Leiner syndrome is due to complement C5 deficiency in infancy and is characterized by seborrhoeic dermatitis, infections, diarrhoea and a failure to thrive.

Lennox–Gastaut syndrome

Lennox–Gastaut syndrome is a common epileptic syndrome which develops in early childhood and is characterized principally by 'absences', in which the child is likely to be damaged by a fall. Other epileptic features are atypical absences, spasms and sometimes myoclonic seizures occurring by day and tonic seizures at night. Intelligence is below average and may decline further. Treatment with sodium valproate has precipitated acute liver failure.

LEOPARD syndrome

LEOPARD syndrome is an autosomal dominant inherited disorder characterized by:

L – lentigenes (freckles) on the head and neck
E – electrocardiographic conduction abnormalities
O – ocular hypertelorism (wide spacing of the eyes)
P – pulmonary stenosis
A – abnormal genitalia
R – retardation of growth
D – deafness, sensorineural.

Other features can be abnormal pigmentation of the iris and retina, subaortic stenosis and hypertrophic cardiomyopathy

Leriche syndrome

Obstruction of the lower end of the abdominal aorta and the aortic bifurcation by thrombosis causes fatigue in the lower limbs, bilateral claudication, pallor and coldness of the feet and legs, and impotence.

Lesch–Nyhan syndrome

Lesch–Nyhan syndrome is an X-linked recessive disorder of male children in which there is a deficiency of the enzyme hypoxanthine-guanine phosphoribosyl transferase. It is characterized by mental retardation, retarded growth, self-mutilation by biting the fingers, lips and tongue, and the development of pyramidal and extrapyramidal signs, with extensor spasm of the trunk, choreoathetosis, dysarthria, exaggerated tendon reflexes and positive Babinski signs. Epileptic seizures are present in about half the patients. Renal failure can occur before puberty. It can be diagnosed *in utero* by assay of hypoxanthine-guanine phosphoribosyl transferase in fetal blood or by the use of an oligonucleotide probe.

Letterer–Siwe syndrome

Other name Schüller–Christian syndrome

Letterer–Siwe syndrome is a form of histiolytic proliferative disease usually presenting in infancy or childhood, occasionally in adult life. Clinical features can include single or multiple eosinophilic granuloma of bone, enlarged lymph nodes, enlarged liver and spleen, pulmonary infiltration, fever, anaemia, thrombocytopenia, mandibular hyperplasia, gingival inflammation and necrosis with loosening and loss of teeth, and cutaneous lesions – papules, vesicles, a moist pruritic lesion of the groin and axillae, a pruritic exudative lesion of the perianal region, vaginal orifice and external auditory meatus and xanthomas. The prognosis for life in childhood is poor but in adults the disease is likely to run a prolonged course.

Lewandowsky–Lutz syndrome

Other name Epidermodysplasia verruciformis

Lewandowsky–Lutz syndrome is a familial disease beginning in early childhood. It is characterized by multiple papillomavirus-induced scaly macules anywhere on the skin and papules on the back of the hand. At 20–30 years lesions which have been exposed to sunlight are likely to develop into Bowen's carcinoma and then into squamous cell carcinoma.

Lewis syndrome

Other name Upper limb cardiovascular syndrome

Lewis syndrome is an autosomal dominant condition in which multiple skeletal abnormalities of the upper limb are associated with congenital heart disease and disturbances of atrial and ventricular cardiac conduction disorders.

Liddle syndrome

Other name Pseudohyperaldosteronism

Liddle syndrome is an autosomal dominant disorder occurring in infancy and characterized by hypertension, hypokalaemic alkalosis and hyperkaliuria with low aldosterone levels. Clinical features include hypertension, headache, retinopathy, abdominal cramp, polyuria, weakness, paralysis and sometimes tetany. Renal function is normal except for the failure to conserve potassium.

Lightwood syndrome

Other name Infantile distal renal tubular acidosis

Lightwood syndrome is a mild and transient form of renal tubular acidosis which appears only in the 1st year of life.

See also Butler–Albright syndrome

Lindau–Hippel syndrome. See Hippel–Landau syndrome

Linear A syndrome

In Linear A syndrome small, itching subepidermal vesicles appear around an erythematous central area on the limbs. On immunopathological examination a fine continuous line of IgA is found at the dermo–epithelial junction.

Lipoprotein lipase deficiency syndrome

Deficiency of lipoprotein lipase (which has a role in triacylglycerol metabolism) causes enlargement of the liver and spleen, abdominal pain, xanthomas and creamy plasma due to an increase in chylomicrons.

Lip pit syndrome

Other name Demarquay syndrome

A familial pit on the lower lip is present and sometimes associated with cleft palate.

Locked-in syndrome

Locked-in syndrome is a syndrome of total paralysis below the level of the third cranial nerve nuclei. The only movements the patient can make are elevation of the eyelids and elevation and depression of the eyes. Consciousness is retained. The causes are infarction of the ventral pons, infarction of efferent motor tracts with preservation of the ascending reticular formation and third cranial nerve nuclei, head injury, brainstem encephalitis, a pontine tumour or haemorrhage, and central pontine myelinosis.

Loeffler syndrome

Other names Pulmonary eosinophilia; perifocal infiltration

Cough, wheezing and fever are due to an eosinophilic infiltration of the lungs. It can occur in asthma or be a reaction to ascaris, microfilaria, *Toxocara canis*, *Toxocara catis* or drugs, such as sodium aminosalicylate.

Longevity syndrome

Longevity syndrome is a mild form of hypercholesterolaemia due to a high level of high density lipoproteins (HDL). It is a benign disorder credited with an increased life expectancy. It can be familial or found in postmenopausal women on hormone replacement therapy or in patients taking phenobarbitone or phenytoin.

Louis-Bar syndrome

Other name Ataxia-telangiectasia

Louis-Bar syndrome is an autosomal recessive disorder characterized by cerebellar ataxia, athetoid movements, nystagmus, slow dysarthric speech, telangiectasia on the conjunctiva and later on the face and limbs, *café au lait* spots, infections of the lungs and ears, hypoplasia of the thymus and spleen, strabismus, bronchiectasis and a progressive mental retardation. The immunoglobulins IgA and IgE are absent and T-cell and B-cell functions are depressed. There is a degeneration of the cerebellar cortex and of sympathetic ganglia and demyelination of the posterior columns of the spinal cord. Affected children usually die before adolescence of a pulmonary infection or a lymphoreticular malignant tumour.

Lowe syndrome

Other name Oculocerebrorenal syndrome

Lowe syndrome is an X-linked recessive disorder characterized by mental retardation, small eyes, congenital cataracts, congenital glaucoma, strabismus, buphthalmos (abnormal enlargement of the eyes), hypotonia, absent tendon reflexes, fits, osteoporosis and a renal tubular defect which causes proteinuria, amine aciduria and acidosis.

Lown–Ganong–Levine syndrome

Lown–Ganong–Levine syndrome is a variation of the Wolff–Parkinson–White syndrome in which the P–R interval is short and the QRS complex is normal: the delta wave is not as obvious as it is in Wolff–Parkinson–White syndrome. It is more common in females. Patients have a high incidence of atrial flutter fibrillation.

Low-pressure syndrome

Low-pressure syndrome is a severe headache lasting for several days following lumbar puncture and due to a persistent leakage of cerebrospinal fluid through the hole in the dura mater.

Low T_3 syndrome. See Euthyroid sick syndrome

Low T_3–T_4 syndrome. See Euthyroid sick syndrome

Lubs syndrome. See Testicular feminization syndrome

Lutembacher syndrome

Lutembacher syndrome can be (a) an atrial septal defect with mitral stenosis, either congenital or due to rheumatic fever, and an enlarged right atrium, or (b) a laceration of the same septum occurring as a complication of mitral valve replacement therapy.

Lyell syndrome

Other name Toxic epidermal necrolysis

Lyell syndrome is a severe bullous eruption of the skin and mucous membranes. Aetiological factors are some drugs (barbiturates, analgesics, hydantoin), bacterial, viral and fungal infections, malignant disease especially lymphoma, vaccinations and radiation. It may be a severe form of erythema multiforme. Clinical features are fever, malaise, conjunctivitis, a diffuse erythema, large bullae developing in the skin and mucous membranes, tracheitis, pneumonia, gastrointestinal haemorrhage, secondary infections, renal impairment and disseminated intravascular coagulation. Recovery is slow and contractures may form in the skin and mucous membranes. There is a high death rate in children and old people.

Lyme syndrome

Lyme syndrome is due to infection by *Borrelia burgdorferi*, a spirochaete transmitted by bites of a tick *Ixodes ricinus*, which has been found on deer, mice, sheep and humans and their pets. It was originally described in children in Old Lyme, Connecticut, USA and has appeared in Britain. A papule appears at the site of the bite and other features appear 3–30 days later. Common clinical features are a rash spreading out from the original papule, low-grade fever, polyarthritis, enlarged lymph nodes in the neck, axillae and groins, headache and fatigue. Untreated, the symptoms and signs can persist for up to 18 months and then gradually disappear. Meningoencephalitis and heart block are uncommon complications.

See also Bannwarth syndrome

M

McArdle syndrome

Other name Muscle phorylase deficiency

Deficiency of muscle phorylase causes stiffness, weakness and muscle pain after exercise. Myoglobinuria can occur.

McCune–Albright syndrome. See Albright syndrome

Macleod syndrome

Other name Swyer–James syndrome

Macleod syndrome is a hypertransradiancy on X-ray of one lung. It can be due to a congenital or acquired pulmonary artery obstruction. It can also occur in children under 5 years of age after pneumonia, and may be associated with Fallot's tetralogy syndrome. Other radiographic features are diminished lung volume, which is more marked on inspiration, a diminished movement of hemidiaphragm, and (especially noted on tomography and arteriography) diminished lung size with a hypoplastic pulmonary artery and branch arteries.

Maffucci syndrome

Other name Kast syndrome

Maffucci syndrome is an association of cavernous haemangiomas, enchondromas (benign tumours of cartilage), anaemia, a labile blood pressure, fragile bones and sensitivity to vasodilator drugs. The haemangiomas are usually in the limbs but they can occur in the retroperitoneal space in the synovial membranes of joints. Complications are pathological fractures, chondrosarcoma and angiosarcoma.

Malabsorption syndrome

Deficiency of proteins, carbohydrates, vitamins and minerals due to steatorrhoea and other causes of malabsorption from the gut can cause loss of weight, diarrhoea, anaemia, dermatitis, moist eczematous skin lesions (mainly in the flexures), oedema, polyneuritis, purpura, bruising and haematuria. It is especially common in elderly people on an inadequate diet.

Malignant carcinoid syndrome

Malignant carcinoid syndrome is due to the secretion of bradykinin and serotonin into the hepatic veins by a secondary carcinoid tumour of the liver. Clinical features are variable. They include evidence of an intra-abdominal malignant tumour, nausea, vomiting, abdominal pain, abdominal distension; flushes, excessive perspiration; dyspnoea, stridor, asthmatic attacks; hypotonia; tachycardia; and later telangiectasia of the face, oedema, arthritis, scleroderma and fibrositis of the valves of the right side of the heart.

Mallory–Weiss syndrome

Mallory–Weiss syndrome is a vomiting-induced tear of the lower end of the oesophagus or of the cardia, with bleeding. It occurs usually in chronic alcoholics.

March syndrome. See Anterior tibial syndrome

Marchesani syndrome

Marchesani syndrome is an autosomal recessive disorder with multiple skeletal and ocular deformities. An affected patient is short and stocky with well developed muscles. The hands and feet are spade shaped. X-rays show delayed carpal and tarsal ossification. The ocular abnormalities include ectopia lentis (displacement of the lens of the eye), spherophakia (a spherical lens), iridodonesis (tremulousness of the iris due to lack of support by the lens) and glaucoma. The prognosis for sight is poor because the glaucoma is unaffected by treatment.

Marchiafava–Bignami syndrome

Marchiafava–Bignami syndrome is a progressive alcoholic syndrome characterized by fits, stupor, coma and dementia. Demyelinating lesions are present in the corpus callosum. It was first described in Italian chianti drinkers.

Marchiafava–Micheli syndrome

Other name Paroxysmal nocturnal haemoglobinuria

Marchiafava–Micheli syndrome is an autoimmune haemolytic anaemia with venous thromboembolism. The excessive red cell destruction takes place mainly at night, and the consequent haemoglobinuria occurs only or mainly in the urine passed on awakening.

Marcus–Gunn syndrome

Other names Gunn syndrome; jaw-winking syndrome

Marcus–Gunn syndrome is a congenital abnormality, probably due to a lesion in the brainstem, in which the upper eyelids are affected by ptosis and are raised whenever the mouth is opened.

Marfan syndrome

Marfan syndrome is an autosomal dominant condition in about three-quarters of affected people; in one quarter it is not inherited but due to a gene mutation. It is a genetic disorder of collagen. Clinical features are asthenic build, tall stature, long arms and legs, arachnodactyly (long spider-like fingers and toes), a highly-arched palate, kyphoscoliosis and easily dislocated joints. Other features can be cataracts, detachment of the retina and dislocation of the lens before the age of 12 years (the suspensory ligaments are at the wrong tension owing to the eyes being too long), aortic regurgitation, mitral regurgitation, coronary thrombosis, dissecting aneurysm of the aorta, pneumothorax, purpura and an often fatal dissecting aneurysm of the aorta. Schizophrenia can be an associated condition.

Marinesco–Sjögren syndrome

Other names Marinesco–Garland syndrome; cataract-oligophrenia syndrome

Marinesco–Sjögren syndrome is an autosomal recessive disorder characterized by cerebellar ataxia, dysarthria, short stature, abnormal teeth, cataracts, brittle thin hair, thin fragile nails and mental retardation.

Marion syndrome

Marion syndrome is an obstruction of the bladder neck in women due to an enlargement of the periurethral glands.

Maroteaux–Lamy syndrome

Other name Mucopolysaccharidosis Type VI

Maroteaux–Lamy syndrome is an autosomal recessive disorder of mucopolysaccharide metabolism due to a deficiency of the enzyme aryl sulphatase B. Clinical features are short stature, lumbar kyphosis, genu valgum, hydrocephalus, valvular disease of the heart and often enlargement of the liver and spleen. Intelligence is normal or near normal. The patient usually survives to the 20s.

Marshall syndrome

Marshall syndrome is an autosomal dominant condition characterized by sensorineural deafness, cataracts and saddle nose.

Masquerade syndromes

Masquerade syndromes are tumours of the eyes which masquerade as uveitis. They can be a lymphoma, a reticulum cell carcinoma, a malignant melanoma, a retinoblastoma or a leukaemic tumour.

Mastocytosis syndrome

Mastocytosis syndrome is a disorder of mast cells, usually beginning in childhood. There is a proliferation of mast cells in many organs (but not in the central nervous system), especially in the skin, liver, spleen, lymph nodes, gastrointestinal tract and bone. Early features are flushing, headache, dizziness, rhinorrhoea, wheezing, nausea, vomiting, diarrhoea, hypotension and sometimes shock. The skin shows localized or generalized pigmented and papular lesions (urticaria pigmentosa) or a generalized flushing with pruritus. Stroking apparently normal skin can cause weals. Other features can be bone pain, enlarged liver and spleen, malabsorption, peptic ulceration, anaemia, leukopenia and thrombocytopenia.

Mayer–Rokitansky–Küster syndrome

Other name Rokitansky–Küster–Haüser syndrome

Mayer–Rokitansky–Küster syndrome is characterized by vaginal aplasia, rudimentary cornua uteri and morphologically-normal ovaries and Fallopian tubes situated on the pelvic side wall. The woman is amenorrhoeic and infertile.

Meadow syndrome. See Munchausen-by-proxy syndrome

Meckel syndrome

Meckel syndrome is an autosomal recessive inherited condition characterized by occipital encephalocele, cataracts, polycystic kidneys, polydactyly, congenital heart disease and abnormal genitalia.

Median arcuate ligament syndrome. See Coeliac artery compression syndrome

Meige syndrome

Meige syndrome is characterized by involuntary facial movements and blepharospasm (spasm of the orbicular muscles), usually presenting in adult life. Speech and swallowing may be interfered with.

Meigs syndrome

Meigs syndrome is a solid ovarian tumour (usually a fibroma) associated with ascites and a pleural effusion.

MELAS syndrome

MELAS syndrome is:

ME – mitochondrial encephalopathy
LA – lactic acidosis
S – stroke-like episodes.

It is a mitochondrial disorder in which can occur ischaemic attacks, prolonged migrainous headaches, attacks of vomiting, partial epileptic seizures, status epilepticus, epilesia partialis continua and cerebral infarctions. As results of these cerebral insults cortical blindness, cortical deafness and dementia develop.

Melkersson–Rosenthal syndrome

Other name Melkersson syndrome

Melkersson–Rosenthal syndrome is characterized by recurrent facial paralysis, oedema of the face and lips and hypertrophy and fissuring of the tongue. The cause is unknown. The paralysis clears up, but the oedema may persist.

Mendelson syndrome

Other names Acid aspiration syndrome; acute exudative pneumonitis

Mendelson syndrome is characterized by cyanosis, bronchospasm and hypotension following the aspiration of the stomach contents into the lungs. It can occur in labour, during anaesthesia late in pregnancy and at other times. The pulmonary epithelium is damaged, with fluid leaking into the alveoli and interstitial spaces. Cardiovascular failure can occur. Pulmonary oedema can cause sudden death or death may occur later from pulmonary complications.

Ménière syndrome

Ménière syndrome is characterized by attacks of vertigo and tinnitus with sensorineural hearing loss. In the early stages of the disease one or two of the symptoms may be present without the third, and the diagnosis should not be made until all three are present. In many patients, the vertigo, tinnitus and hearing loss are similar to those produced by hydrops of the labyrinth.

Menkes syndrome

Other name Kinky hair disease

Menkes syndrome is an inherited recessive disorder associated with a copper enzyme deficiency state. Clinical features are sparse kinky hair, seborrhoeic dermatitis, hypopigmentation and neurological retardation. Death from central nervous system complications can occur before 2 years of age.

MERRF syndrome

MERRF syndrome is a disorder of mitochondrial metabolism characterized by:

ME – myoclonic epilepsy
RRF – ragged-red muscle fibres.

Mesenteric artery syndrome

Vomiting and other features of intestinal obstruction occur in childhood said to be due to an obstruction of the duodenum by an angulation of the superior mesenteric artery, which seems unlikely.

Mesenteric steal syndrome

If the coeliac artery is obstructed, the blood to the hepatic and splenic arteries has to pass through the superior mesenteric artery, the inferior pancreaticoduodenal artery and the gastroduodeneal artery. It is usually asymptomatic, but the small bowel may be deprived of blood and this can cause postprandial 'abdominal angina'.

Meyer–Kouwenaar syndrome

Meyer–Kouwenaar syndrome is a form of filiariasis in which massive eosinophilia is associated with enlargement of the lymph nodes, liver and spleen.

Mikulicz syndrome

Other name Uveoparotid syndrome

Chronic dacryoadenitis with lacrimal gland enlargement is associated with enlargement of the salivary glands. It can be self-limiting or it can occur in tuberculosis, sarcoidosis, lymphatic leukaemia or lymphosarcoma.

Middle aortic syndrome

Middle aortic syndrome is a congenital narrowing of the aorta proximal to the renal arteries and other visceral branches. It is more common in boys than girls.

Middle lobe syndrome. See Brock syndrome

Mieten syndrome

Mieten syndrome is an autosomal recessive disorder characterized by short stature, short forearms, dislocation of the radius, flexion contracture of the elbow, strabismus and mental retardation.

Milk-alkali syndrome

Milk-alkali syndrome is hypercalcaemia due to consumption by peptic ulcer patients of excessive amounts of alkalis over a long period of time. It can also be caused by secondary or tertiary hyperparathyroidism, due to a chronic reduction of ionized calcium. An elevated parathyroid hormone concentration which returned to normal with conservative treatment has also been reported.

Milkman syndrome

Milkman syndrome is characterized by osteoporosis with multiple patho-logical fractures and occurs usually in middle-aged women.

Millard–Gubler syndrome

Other name Millard–Gubler–Foville syndrome

Millard–Gubler syndrome is similar to Foville syndrome, but as the lesion is lower in the pons it misses the supranuclear pathway for conjugate lateral gaze. The clinical features are a crossed hemiplegia and ipsilateral paralysis of the abducens and facial nerves, without a horizontal gaze paralysis.

Miller–Dieker syndrome

Miller–Dieker syndrome is one of the contiguous syndromes in which there is a combination of mental retardation and physical malformations. In this syndrome there is a deletion on chromosome 17, detectable by gene mapping or the use of restriction fragment length polymorphs.

Minimal change nephrotic syndrome. See Nephrotic syndrome

Mixed ataxic and spastic syndrome

Spasticity and ataxia affecting one or more limbs can be due to a lesion in the brainstem involving the cerebellar pathways and the descending long tract pathways. Such a syndrome can occur in multiple sclerosis.

Möbius syndrome

Möbius syndrome is an autosomal dominant condition characterized by bilateral paralysis of the sixth and seventh cranial nerves, deafness, stra-bismus, ptosis, muscular weakness of the neck, chest and tongue, and difficulties in chewing and swallowing.

Moersch–Woltmann syndrome. See Stiff man syndrome

Mononeuritis multiplex syndrome

Mononeuritis multiplex syndrome is the occurrence of several acute and often painful neuropathies developing at different sites of the body and at about the same time. They can be due to the pressure effects on different plexuses, roots and nerves, but they are more likely to be due to vascular lesions of the nerves in generalized disorders. These disorders can be arteritis, cancer, diabetes mellitus, leprosy, paraproteinaemias, polyarteritis nodosa, sarcoidosis, systemic lupus erythematosus, Wegener's granulomatosis and intravenous drugs abuse.

Morquio syndrome

Other name Mucopolysaccharidosis Type IV

Morquio syndrome is an autosomal recessive inherited disorder of mucopolysaccharides. In the A form there is a deficiency of the enzyme galactosamine-6-sulphate sulphatase; in the B form there is a deficiency of the enzyme β-galactosidase. Clinical features are short stature, coarse features, prominent sternum, kyphosis, genu valgum, waddling gait and corneal opacities. Aortic incompetence can develop later in life. Intelligence may be below average. In the B form the bone changes are slight; the odontoid process of the second cervical vertebra may be aplastic. The deformities are likely to become progressively worse. Most patients survive to early adulthood. Death may be due to cervical dislocation.

Morris syndrome. See Testicular feminization syndrome

Moschcowitz syndrome

Other name Thrombotic thrombocytopenic purpura

Moschcowitz syndrome is a fulminating and often fatal syndrome and it is characterized by thrombocytopenia, thromboses, purpura, haemolytic anaemia, renal failure and neurological symptoms.

Mounier–Kuhn syndrome

Other name Tracheobronchomegaly

Mounier–Kuhn syndrome is a congenital enlargement of the trachea and bronchi. The trachea can be 35–50 mm in diameter. It leads to attacks of bronchitis, bronchiolitis, pneumonia, emphysema, bronchiectasis and pulmonary fibrosis. It may be associated with Ehlers–Danlos syndrome.

Moynahan syndrome

Moynahan syndrome is a congenital disorder characterized by multiple symmetrical lentigenes (freckles), congenital mitral stenosis and short stature.

Muckle–Wells syndrome

Muckle–Wells syndrome is an autosomal dominant inherited condition of amyloidosis (especially of the kidneys), deafness, and febrile attacks with muscle pain and urticaria.

Mucocutaneous lymph node syndrome

Other name Kawasaki disease

Mucocutaneous lymph node syndrome is a disease of unknown origin characterized by generalized lymphadenopathy with fever, conjunctivitis, pharyngitis, erythema of the hands and feet, arthritis, proteinuria and arterial aneurysms, especially of the coronary arteries. It usually affects young children.

Mucosal neuroma syndrome

Other name Multiple endocrine neoplasia Type III

Mucosal neuroma syndrome may be a variant of Sipple syndrome (multiple endocrine neoplasia Type II). Clinical features include neuromas of the mouth, nose, upper gastrointestinal tract and conjunctiva associated with phaeochromocytoma and medullary thyroid carcinoma. Other features can be lentigenes (freckles), *cafe au lait* spots on the skin, 'blubbery lips', lax joints, kyphoscoliosis, diverticulosis and megacolon. Death is usually due to medullary thyroid carcinoma.

Muir–Torre syndrome

Muir–Torre syndrome is an inherited condition (probably autosomal dominant) characterized by sebaceous tumours of the skin associated with multiple visceral tumours, usually of the gastrointestinal tract.

Multiple endocrine adenoma syndrome

Other name Pluriglandular adenomas

Multiple endocrine adenoma syndrome is an association, often familial, of several endocrine tumours in one patient, especially (Type 1) parathyroid tumour, pancreatic islet tumour, pituitary tumour and (Type 2) parathyroid tumour, thyroid tumour, adrenal medullary tumour.

Multiple hamartoma syndrome

Other name Cowden syndrome

Multiple hamartoma syndrome is a familial disorder characterized by multiple hamartomas (benign tumour-like nodules) and a 'cobblestone' appearance of the mucosa membranes, which have papules in them. Associated features are small jaws, scoliosis, thyroid adenoma, breast hypertrophy, fibrocystic disease or cancer.

Cowden was the name of the family in which it was first described.

Multiple organ failure syndrome

Multiple organ failure syndrome is failure of the heart, liver, kidneys and other organs due to severe sepsis, trauma, burns and major surgery.

Multiple vertebral compression-fracture syndrome

Multiple vertebral compression-fracture syndrome is characterized by severe and disabling compression fractures of several vertebral bodies due to osteoporosis induced by corticosteroids.

Munchausen syndrome

Other names Hospital addiction; chronic factitious illness; hospital hobo

Munchausen syndrome is a syndrome in which a vagrant repeatedly seeks hospital admission by faking the symptoms of an acute abdominal or other illness and, if admitted, he may endure investigations and operation: having been discharged he is likely to turn up at another hospital with the same story, or at the original hospital with another story. Epileptic seizures, status epilepticus, meningitis, coronary thrombosis and mental illness can also be mimicked. The man (it can be a woman) differs from a malingerer in that he does not fake illness to avoid work or to get money but does it for varied psychological reasons.

It is an ill-named syndrome. Baron Karl Munchausen (1720–97) was a German soldier of fortune who, on his return from the wars, would relate fantastic and, probably, fictitious accounts of his adventures, which were afterwards put down in a book. Munchausen was probably a pathological liar, but he did not exhibit the syndrome to which his name has been given. It might more accurately have been called 'Simulated sickness syndrome'.

See also Munchausen-mammae syndrome; Munchausen-by-proxy syndrome

Munchausen-by-proxy syndrome

Other name Meadow syndrome

In Munchausen-by-proxy syndrome a mother ascribes to her children illnesses that they do not have. Epilepsy is the commonest. In the 'active'

form she induces anoxia and seizures by suffocating the child for a few moments, as by pressing the child's face hard against her bosom. In the 'passive' form she complains or teaches the children to complain that the child experiences fits or other conditions such as diarrhoea, abdominal colic, haematemesis, haematuria or apnoeic attacks. Children may be admitted to hospital, intensively investigated and treated with anticonvulsants before the correct diagnosis is made. Children who have been brought up in this way can take over the illness pattern themselves and lead a life of invalidism or repeatedly present themselves to hospital with stories of imaginary illness (like a vagrant with Munchausen syndrome).
See also Munchausen syndrome

Munchausen-mammae syndrome

A woman with normal breasts and without symptoms who demands over-frequent examination of her breasts clinically and by radiology or sonamammography.
See also Munchausen syndrome

Mutism-anarthritic syndrome

Mutism-anarthritic syndrome is one of the 'lacunar' syndromes in which lacunae (small spaces) in the internal capsules cause dysarthria (imperfect articulation) and anarthria (severe dysarthria resulting in mutism). It can progress to the pseudobulbar syndrome.

Myasthenic syndrome. See Eaton–Lambert syndrome

Myelodysplastic syndrome

Myelodysplastic syndrome is a heterogenous group of haemopoietic disorders characterized by cytopenia, despite a normal cellular bone marrow, due to the gradual expansion of an abnormal haemopoietic stem cell clone. An infection can be fatal.

Myofascial pain syndrome

Other name Fibrositis

Myofascial pain syndrome is characterized by chronic aches and pain and stiffness in many parts of the body – muscles, joints, tendon insertions, ligaments, subcutaneous tissues and bony prominences – with trigger (tendon) points of localized increased tenderness. Sleep is often disturbed.

N

Naegeli syndrome. See Francheschetti–Jodassohn syndrome

Naevus sebaceous syndrome

Naevus sebaceous syndrome is one of the neuroectodermal syndromes. It is characterized by yellow-orange coloured linear lesions in the skin of the forehead and midface area. The cause is unknown.

Naffziger syndrome. See Scalenus syndrome

Nail-patella syndrome

Other names Turner–Kieser syndrome; hereditary onycho-osteodysplasia

In this autosomal dominant disorder the patella is small or absent and the nails show changes varying from ridging to absence; the thumb nails are the ones usually affected. Other anomalies may be exostoses of the ileum, malformed radial heads and pigmentary changes in the iris. Of all sufferers from this syndrome, 40% develop renal disease, and of those 25% progress to renal failure.

NAME syndrome

NAME syndrome is characterized by:

N – naevi
A – atrial myxoma
M – myxoid neurofibromas
E – ephelides (freckles)

It may be the same as LAMB syndrome

Nance–Horan syndrome

Nance–Horan syndrome is a X-linked congenital condition characterized by cataracts, peg-shaped and supernumerary teeth, and in about 20% of cases broad or short fingers, developmental delay, and mental retardation.

Narcoleptic syndrome

This condition is characterized by narcolepsy (a recurrent uncontrollable desire for sleep, with sleep not usually lasting more than 20 minutes), cataplexy (a sudden loss of postural tone without loss of consciousness), sleep paralysis (short periods of inability to move on either falling asleep or awakening) and dream-like vivid hallucinations.

Near-miss sudden infant death syndrome

Near-miss sudden infant death syndrome describes an infant who is found lying apparently unconscious, not breathing, cyanotic or pale, limp and in need of stimulation or mouth-to-mouth resuscitation as death seems imminent. The child has previously been normal and with no history of fever or fits. While some of these infants may be developing an infective, traumatic, metabolic or other illness, for others there is no explanation. Gastro-oesophageal reflux is a possible factor, and there is a possibility that the mother may have deliberately suffocated the child. Some infants do not regain consciousness and they die. Survivors can develop a hypoxic-ischaemic encephalopathy, coma, status epilepticus, brainstem dysfunction and cortical blindness.

See also Sudden infant death syndrome; Munchausen-by-proxy syndrome

Nelson syndrome I

An adrenocorticotrophic hormone (ACTH)-secreting tumour of the pituitary gland, which is locally invasive, causing severe defects of the visual fields. Hyperpigmentation of the skin due to ACTH or β-lipotropin hypersecretion usually occurs.

Nelson syndrome II

Nelson syndrome II is an association of a hair defect (in which the distal ends of the hairs are invaginated into the proximal ends, giving them a bamboo-like appearance) with icthyosis linearis circumflexa (a multicyclic eruption, diffuse erythema and scaling).

Neonatal lupus syndrome

Neonatal lupus syndrome is characterized by cutaneous lupus or congenital heart block in a neonate whose mother has a connective tissue disease (such as systemic lupus erythematosus or Sjögren syndrome) and/or has the autoantibodies anti-Ro, anti-La or anti-U1 RNP. The cutaneous lupus may be present at birth or develop within 5 months. The heart block develops abruptly during the later weeks of pregnancy and is permanent.

Other cardiovascular anomalies can be other conduction anomalies, patent ductus arteriosus and myocarditis. Death in the perinatal period is common, but survival up to adulthood can occur, with most patients requiring a pacemaker before the age of 50.

Nephrotic syndrome

Other names Minimal change nephrotic syndrome; lipid nephrosis

Nephrotic syndrome is characterized by severe proteinuria, oedema, hypoalbuminaemia and hyperlipidaemia. It can follow any disease involving the glomeruli. In children it usually follows minimal change disease or a viral infection; in adults it usually follows membranous glomerulonephritis. The oedema begins in the periorbital regions and quickly becomes generalized. The cause of the hyperlipidaemia is not clear: possibly very low density lipoprotein (VLDL) synthesis is increased because the hypoalbuminaemia causes fatty acids to be taken up more easily by the liver. The hyperlipidaemia does not cause atheroma. Complications are pleural effusion, ascites, renal vein thrombosis, renal function impairment and infections, especially pneumococcal peritonitis in children.

See also Congenital nephrotic syndrome

Neuroectodermal syndromes

This term includes the following neuroectodermal disorders: focal dermal hypoplasia (focal atrophy of the skin, irregular patches of pigmentation in the skin, lipomatous nodules); hypomelanosis of Ito (patches of hypopigmentation on the trunk and limbs); incontinentia pigmenti (blisters at birth, followed by patches of hyperpigmentation); naevus sebaceous syndrome; neurofibromatosis (subcutaneous neurofibromas, *café au lait* spots in the skin); Sturge–Weber syndrome and tuberous sclerosis (adenoma sebaceum, shagreen patches, hypopigmented macules, severe mental retardation).

Neuroleptic malignant syndrome

Other name Supersensitivity syndrome

Neuroleptic malignant syndrome is a severe and life-threatening reaction to antipsychotic drugs (such as haloperidol, chlorpromazine, trifluoperazine, lithium, thioridazine, sulpiride, zuclopenthixol decanoate, metoclopramide, carbamazepine). It is characterized by hyperpyrexia, rapid respiration, drowsiness, restlessness and parkinsonism. Associated conditions are renal failure and rhabdomyolosis (death of striated muscle with excretion of myoglobin in the urine) and myoglobinaemia. It occurs very rapidly and the full syndrome can be present within 48 hours of the appearance of the first symptom. The serum creatinine phosphokinase is increased by the muscle breakdown. It is a potentially malignant syndrome, but with treatment a fatal outcome is unusual.

A similar condition, but without parkinsonian rigidity, has been reported in cocaine abuse.

Newborn withdrawal syndrome

Newborn withdrawal syndrome can occur in newly born babies whose mothers have taken narcotic drugs during pregnancy or were drug addicts. Clinical features are a reduction of fetal functions and growth, apnoeic attacks, respiratory depression, hypothermia, hypotonia and tachycardia. The babies of drug addicts are particularly at risk and are likely to show the features of the syndrome to a severe degree and may also have gastrointestinal and central nervous system disorders with a possibility of perinatal death. When cocaine has been the drug, the baby can also show irritability and EEG abnormalities which resolve in time.

Nezelof syndrome

Other name Combined immunodeficiency with predominant T-cell defect

Nezelof syndrome is a form of immunodeficiency with absent or few T cells, dysplasia of the thymus, skin rashes, failure to thrive and severe infections with low resistance to them. B cells and serum immunoglobins are normal. It has occurred in children with congenital viral infections, such as cytomegalovirus infection. The long-term prognosis is poor.

Nocturnal myoclonus syndrome

Nocturnal myoclonus syndrome is characterized by short bouts of myoclonus occurring at night and restlessness of the legs, sometimes associated with attacks of sleep by day.

No-maybe-sometimes-yes syndrome

No-maybe-sometimes-yes syndrome is the hesitant admission by a frightened or mentally blocked young child when being interviewed because he or she is thought to have been sexually abused.

Noonan syndrome

The patient with Noonan syndrome resembles a patient with Turner syndrome, but there is no chromosomal defect and Noonan syndrome occurs in both sexes. Clinical features are intelligence below average, short stature, low-set ears and many minor skeletal deformities of which the commonest are pectus excavatum and cubitus valgus. Cardiac abnormalities occur in 50% of patients: these include pulmonary valve stenosis, thick and dysplastic pulmonary valves, right heart anomalies and left ventricular cardiomyopathy.

Norrie syndrome

Norrie syndrome is an X-linked form of congenital blindness, with a pseudotumour of the retina, leukokoria (white appearance of the pupil) and progressive mental deterioration.

Nothnagel syndrome

Nothnagel syndrome is characterized by ocular paralyses, paralysis of gaze, and cerebellar ataxia, due to a tumour involving the superior cerebellar peduncles.

Numb chin syndrome

In numb chin syndrome, numbness of the chin is due to an isolated mental nerve palsy. It can be the result of trauma, drug toxicity or a tumour of the jaw. In old people it can be due to atrophy of the mandible. It was first described by Charles Bell (of Bell's palsy fame).

Occipital lobe syndromes

Lesions of an occipital lobe can be an infarction, a tumour or a degenerative disease of the brain. A lesion is likely to cause visual field defects. A lesion of the anterior part of a lobe can cause a disorder of visual perception without there being any visual impairment; the patient may be unable to recognize faces. Other syndromes that can be produced are Anton syndrome and visual agnosia syndrome. Bilateral lesions can cause total blindness.

Oculocerebral-hypopigmentation syndrome. See Cross–McKusick–Breen syndrome

Oculocerebrorenal syndrome. See Lowe syndrome

Oculocraniosomatic syndrome

Oculocraniosomatic syndrome is a form of muscular dystrophy characterized by cerebellar ataxia, deafness, heart block, corticospinal signs and retinitis pigmentosa. Muscle biopsy shows ragged-red fibres which suggest that there is a mitochondrial myopathy.

Oculodentodigital syndrome

Oculodentodigital syndrome is characterized by glaucoma, hypoplastic tooth enamel and abnormal digits. Associated features can be sensorineural deafness, cleft lip and palate and congenital dislocation of the hip.

OKT3 syndrome

Fever, headache and confusion due to a mild and self-limiting meningoencephalitis can be induced by OKT3, a monoclonal antibody used to treat threatened rejection of an organ transplant.

Ollier syndrome

Other name Chondrodysplasia

In Ollier syndrome multiple islets of unossified cartilage remain in the shafts of long bones. They are usually bilateral but not symmetrical. Shortness of a limb can occur and sometimes a tumour can be felt in the bone.

Olmstead syndrome

Other name Mutilating palmoplantar keratoderma with periorifacial keratotic plaques

Olmstead syndrome is a form of hereditary palmoplantar keratoma with progressive and disabling palmoplantar keratoderma (horny growths) with hyperkeratotic plaques around the mouth and nostrils.

Omenn syndrome

Omenn syndrome is reticuloendotheliosis associated with eosinophilia.

One-and-a-half syndrome

One-and-a-half syndrome is due to damage of the pontine reticular system, which causes (a) paralysis of all conjugate lateral eye movement ('one') ipsilateral to the lesion, and (b) ipsilateral internuclear ophthalmoplegia ('and-a-half'), including adduction paralysis in the ipsilateral eye and abduction nystagmus in the contralateral eye.

Opitz–Frias syndrome

Other names G syndrome; hypospadias-dysphagia syndrome

Opitz–Frias syndrome is a congenital disorder characterized by craniofacial abnormalities, genital abnormalities, achalasia of the cardia, laryngeal hypoplasia and functional swallowing and laryngeal difficulties. Pulmonary aspiration can occur frequently and be fatal. Males are more severely affected than females. It can present difficulties for an anaesthetist.

Oppenheim syndrome

Other name Useless hand of Oppenheim

Oppenheim syndrome is characterized by clumsiness and uselessness of the hands due to multiple sclerosis affecting the lateral limits of the posterior columns of the spinal cord in the cervical region.

132

Oral dysaesthesia complex syndrome

Swelling and burning of the lips in an elderly patient are associated with a dry mouth, burning of the tongue, a bad taste and sometimes 'stringy' saliva.

Oro-oculo-genital syndrome

Other name Riboflavin deficiency

Deficiency of riboflavin (vitamin B_2) causes a condition resembling pellagra, beginning with pallor of the mucosa at the angles of the mouth, followed by maceration and moist linear fissures. The skin of the nose, ears and eyelids becomes greasy and scaly. Other features can be an angular blepharitis, angular stomatitis, glossitis with the tongue of a magenta colour, white angular lesions (perlèche) in the oral mucosa, corneal vascularization and lesions of the vulva or scrotum. The Plummer–Vinson syndrome may be present.

Osler–Weber–Rendu syndrome

Other name Hereditary haemorrhagic telangiectasia

Osler–Weber–Rendu syndrome is an autosomal dominant condition characterized by telangiectasia of the skin and of the oral, nasal and gastrointestinal mucous membranes. They are liable to ulcerate and bleed. Epistaxis and gastrointestinal haemorrhages are common features. Bleeding may be difficult to control, although clotting factors are normal. Vascular malformations may also be present in the lungs, liver and central nervous system.

Othello syndrome

Othello syndrome is a persistent delusion that the spouse is unfaithful, a delusion that can lead to murder. It can occur in paranoid schizophrenia, paranoid states and severe personality disorder.

Otopalatal digital syndrome

Otopalatal digital syndrome is a recessive inherited condition characterized by short stature, cleft palate, deafness, frontal bossing, hypertelorism (wide spacing of the eyes) and a short broad thumb and toes. In females the features appear in a less marked form.

Ovarian hyperstimulation syndrome

Ovarian hyperstimulation syndrome is due to excessive stimulation of the ovaries by clomiphene citrate and gonadotrophin releasing hormone given in the treatment of female infertility. Induction of ovulation is followed by clinical features of varying degree. Mild hyperstimulation (ovarian enlargement up to 5 cm) can cause mild abdominal discomfort. Moderate hyperstimulation (ovarian enlargement 5–12 cm) can cause abdominal discomfort, nausea and vomiting. Severe hyperstimulation (ovarian enlargement more than 12 cm) is a serious condition with ascites, pleural effusion, electrolyte imbalance, haemoconcentration, hypercoagulability, and oliguria. Complications are severe respiratory embarrassment, disseminated intravascular coagulation, thromboembolism, and renal failure – any one of which can be fatal. The enlarged cysts can be easily ruptured.

Overfeeding syndrome

Other name Intravenous hyperalimentation

Overfeeding syndrome can occur as a complication of total parenteral nutrition. Undesirable metabolic changes can occur if a severely stressed patient or a malnourished patient is administered parenterally calories in excess of metabolic need or is given glucose without fat calories in quantatively important amounts. The administration of more calories than are needed leads to storage of fat.

Overuse syndromes

There are two types.

1. Pain and loss of function in muscle groups and tendons can be due to excessive use by such people as musicians and typists who have to make rapid precise movements of the fingers over a long time. It may cause them to give up their work permanently. In schoolchildren and adolescents it can be due to excessive sports activities, producing such conditions as tennis elbow and, in the United States, 'Little League shoulder'.

2. There can be a general feeling of malaise, with or without orthopaedic problems, experienced by spinal cord injury patients who have engaged in prolonged wheelchair-type exercises.

P

Paediatric concussion syndrome

Concussion in infants and young children is characterized by a deterioration in consciousness minutes or hours after an apparently mild head injury. Other features can be irritability, pallor, vomiting, slight ataxia and sleepiness. The child recovers in a few hours.

Painful bruising syndrome. See Gardner–Diamond syndrome

Pancoast syndrome

Pain in the arm associated with Horner syndrome is due to an invasion of the brachial plexus and cervical lymphatic chain by a bronchial carcinoma of the lung apex.

Papillon–Lefèvre syndrome

Other name Hyperkeratosis palmoplantaris and premature periodontoclasia

Papillon–Lefèvre syndrome is an autosomal recessive disorder presenting in the first 6 months of life. Hyperkeratosis of the palms and soles is associated with later premature loss of deciduous and permanent teeth.

Papillon–Psaume syndrome

Papillon–Psaume syndrome is an autosomal dominant condition characterized by microcephaly, malformed canthi of the eye, defective alar cartilage of the nose, webbed fingers, tremor, frontal alopecia, defects of the lip and palate with normal or below average growth. It is lethal to males: only females survive.

Parachute mitral valve syndrome. See Shone syndrome

Paralytic shellfish syndrome

Paralytic shellfish syndrome is due to eating shellfish contaminated by a toxin produced by red algae (*Dinoflagellata gonyaulax*). Clinical features are numbness of the face, tingling of fingers and paralysis of muscles which, if it reaches the diaphragm, can be fatal.

Parietal lobe syndromes

Parietal lobe lesions, usually an infarction or a tumour, can cause various symptoms and signs, some of which occur with both the dominant and the non-dominant lobe.

Common effects are contralateral hemisensory disturbances, such as astereognosis (an inability to recognize objects by feeling them) and agraphaesthesia (an inability to recognize written and printed letters and words). Lesions of the dominant lobe also cause dysphasia (lack of co-ordination in speech and an inability to put words in their proper order), bilateral apraxia (inability to perform purposeful movements), disorder of language, especially alexia (an inability to read) and Gerstmann syndrome. A lesion of the non-dominant lobe can cause disorder of the body image, such as that half the body is thought to be missing or a paralysed limb is totally ignored, dressing apraxia (inability to dress oneself), and topo-graphical agnosia (an inability to appreciate where one is or recognize previously known places).

Parinaud syndrome

Other name Oculoglandular syndrome

Parinaud syndrome is characterized by paralysis of gaze in a vertical plane, usually associated with dilatation of the pupil, loss of convergence, loss of pupillary accommodation reflex, and sometimes with nystagmus, ptosis or lid retraction, papilloedema or third cranial nerve palsy. It can be due to a vascular lesion, trauma, an infiltrating glioma or a pinealoma in the periaqueductal area.

Patau syndrome

Other name Trisomy 13 syndrome

Multiple abnormalities are produced by trisomy of chromosome number 13. These abnormalities include scalp defects, coloboma (absence of part of the iris, choroid coat or other part of the eye), hypertelorism (wide spacing of the eyes), cleft lip, cleft palate, deformed ears, congenital heart disease, an abnormal thumb, hydronephrosis, hydroureter, bicornate uterus and mental retardation. Death usually occurs before 1 year of life is achieved.

Paterson–Kelly syndrome. See Plummer–Vinson syndrome

Pearlman syndrome

Pearlman syndrome is a familial (probably autosomal recessive) condition characterized by fetal gigantism, renal abnormalities, mental retardation, hyperplasia of the endocrine pancreas which can cause hyperinsulinaemia and hypoglycaemia, and multiple minor abnormalities. Wilms' tumour can develop in childhood. Apnoeic spells can occur.

Pelizaeus–Merzbacher syndrome

Other name Aplasia axialis extracorticalis congenita

Pelizaeus–Merzbacher syndrome is an X-linked diffuse cerebral sclerosis of infancy producing involuntary movements of the head and eyes, nystagmus, spasticity and dementia.

Pendred syndrome

Pendred syndrome is an autosomal recessive disorder of thyroid biosynthesis with a goitre and nerve deafness in childhood.

Pepper syndrome

Pepper syndrome is a neuroblastoma of the adrenal gland with metastases in the liver. It was formerly believed that tumours of the right adrenal had metastases in the liver and tumours of the left adrenal had metastases in the skull.

Periodic syndrome

Periodic syndrome is characterized by attacks of vomiting, abdominal pain, headache and joint pains in childhood, without organic origin and an expression of anxiety or of a communication dysfunction in which the child is not able to put his feelings into words.

Peutz–Jeghers syndrome

Peutz–Jeghers syndrome is an autosomal dominant condition characterized by gastrointestinal polyposis (especially of the small intestine) associated with lentigenes (freckles) around the lips and oral pigmentation. Abdominal pain can occur and pigmentation on the arms and legs. Complications are intussusception caused by a polyp, melaena due to bleeding from a polyp, ovarian neoplasms in affected women and, rarely, malignant

PHC syndrome. See Böök syndrome

Pickwickian syndrome

Other name Cardiorespiratory syndrome of obesity

Pickwickian syndrome is characterized by extreme obesity, mechanical obstruction to pulmonary ventilation, hypoxia, hypercapnia, secondary erythrocytocis (raised red-cell count, haemoglobin concentration and packed cell volume), intense diurnal somnolence and cardiac failure.

PIE syndrome. Pulmonary infiltrate-eosinophilia. See Loeffler syndrome

Piebald syndrome

In piebald syndrome, which is usually transmitted as an autosomal dominant, there is an absence of melanocytes in parts of the skin in a neonate. The skin has a piebald appearance as patches of the skin are white because of a complete absence of pigment cells whilst the rest of the skin is normal colour.

Pierre Robin syndrome

Other name First and second arch syndrome

Pierre Robin syndrome is an autosomal dominant condition characterized by multiple abnormalities, including a hypoplastic mandible and receding chin, glaucoma, cataract, sensorineural deafness, posterior displacement of the tongue (which obstructs breathing and can be an anaesthetic hazard), cleft soft and hard palate without cleft of the lip, a small epiglottis and abnormalities of the fingers and toes. Intelligence may be normal or low. The gag reflex can be absent and attacks of choking and cyanosis can occur.

Pigment dispersion syndrome

Pigment dispersion syndrome is a disorder of the eye in which pigment from the iris is deposited on the corneal epithelium and in the trabecular meshwork of the ciliary body, causing a rise in intraocular pressure. The iris looks atrophic.

Pill depression syndrome

Pill depression syndrome is depression as a side-effect of oral contraceptives. Some cases are thought to be due to pyridoxine deficiencies, probably induced by oestrogen in the pill.

Plummer–Vinson syndrome

Other name Paterson–Kelly syndrome; sideropenic dysphagia

Plummer–Vinson syndrome is characterized by an iron-deficiency anaemia, atrophic glossitis, koilonycha (spoon-shaped finger nails), and dysphagia. It is most common in middle-aged women. The dysphagia is due to a web formed in the postcricoid region. Carcinoma of the tongue and postcricoid region are complications.

The syndrome is also seen in sideropenia (reduced serum iron without evidence of anaemia).

POEMS syndrome

POEMS syndrome is a plasma cell dyscrasia characterized by:

P – polyneuropathy
O – organomegaly (enlarged liver, spleen, lymph nodes)
E – endocrinopathy (hyperthyroidism, diabetes mellitus)
M – monoclonal gammopathy
S – skin changes (hyperpigmentation, hirsutism, thickening, excessive sweating).

Poland syndrome

Poland syndrome is a group of unilateral congenital anomalies of the chest wall with or without involvement of the arm on the same side. The right side is affected twice as often as the left side and there is a 3:1 male:female predominance. The commonest abnormality is absence of the pectoralis major and minor muscles. Syndactyly with absence of the sternal head of pectoralis major can occur.

Polyangiitis overlap syndrome

Polyangiitis overlap syndrome is a form of systemic vasculitis which has overlapping features of several forms of vasculitis (polyarteritis nodosa, Churg–Strauss syndrome, hypersensitivity vasculitis, Henoch–Schönlein purpura, Takayasu's arteritis, temporal arteritis, Wegener's granulomatosis) but does not clinically conform to any one of them. Clinical features can include necrotizing vasculitis in the skin, lung and muscle, pulmonary infiltrates, asthma, eosinophilia, glomerulonephritis, temporal arteritis, venulitis of the skin, vasculitis of small vessels, coronary artery disease, aneurysms of hepatic and renal vessels, and aortic arch disease.

Polycystic ovarian syndrome

Other name Stein–Leventhal syndrome

Polycystic ovarian syndrome is characterized by multiple ovarian cysts, obesity, hirsutism, amenorrhoea or oligomenorrhoea, infertility and sometimes hyperprolactinaemia and virilization. Acne and an increased sebaceous gland activity can be present. Androgen production by the ovaries is increased and there are high levels of plasma testosterone.

Polysplenia syndrome

Polysplenia syndrome is characterized by multiple small spleens in the right and left side of the abdomen and occasionally in the midline. Associated conditions can be transposition of the liver and spleen, malrotation of the bowel, absence of the gallbladder, dextrocardia, congenital heart disease, abnormalities of the great veins, and bilateral bilobed lungs.

Pontine syndrome

Lesions of the pons can cause paralysis of the seventh (facial) cranial nerve (with paralysis of the muscles of the face), the sixth (abducens) cranial nerve (with paralysis of the lateral rectus muscle of the eyeball) and paralysis of the motor part of the fifth (trigeminal) cranial nerve (with paralysis of the muscles of mastication). The lesion is likely to be an infarction or a tumour.

Popliteal web syndrome

Popliteal web syndrome is an inherited syndrome characterized by popliteal and other webs, syndactyly, absent or defective teeth, absent eyebrows and lashes, sparse brittle short scalp hair and toe-nail dysplasia.

Posne–Schlossman syndrome

Other name Acute glaucomatocyclitic crisis

Posne–Schlossman syndrome is characterized by intermittent attacks of acute rises in intraocular pressure, associated with mild anterior uveitis affecting one eye in young adults. Vision is blurred and the pupil dilated. An attack usually lasts for a few hours, but it can last much longer. A colour change can develop in the affected iris. The aetiology is unknown.

Postablation syndrome

Postablation syndrome is fever, pain, haematuria and leukocytosis following ablation of the renal artery (which can be performed to control haemorrhage, reduce pain, reduce the size of tumours or increase immunity).

Postcardiotomy syndrome. See Cardiotomy syndrome

Postcholecystectomy syndrome

Postcholecystectectomy syndrome is characterized by recurrent abdominal pain in the right upper quadrant of the abdomen after a cholecystectomy due to gallstones inadvertently left behind or which have re-formed in the bile ducts, which can occur if there is a stricture of the bile ducts causing stasis or if there is a metabolic abnormality with excretion of an excessive amount of bile pigments.

Postconcussional syndrome

Other name Post-trauma syndrome

Postconcussional syndrome is characterized by headache, dizziness, fatigue and psychological disturbances following a head injury, which is usually a minor one. It is uncommon after an injury in sport and most common in people who are claiming compensation for the injury, and there may be a large element of malingering in their symptoms.

Posterior column syndrome

Lesions of the posterior column of the spinal cord cause loss of position sense and vibration sense with preservation of touch, pain and temperature senses. Pins-and-needles and tingling are common. The hands and feet feel swollen at night. When the sensory loss affects the legs the patient can have a sensory ataxia and positive Romberg reaction. Sensory loss in the hands produces an inability to recognize coins in a bag or pocket and difficulty in handling small objects.

Postgastrectomy syndrome

The sequelae of partial gastrectomy can be a feeling of fullness after meals (due to the smaller stomach size), dumping, diarrhoea and bilious vomiting due to kinking or obstruction of the afferent loop. An iron-deficiency anaemia can be associated, due to loss of or reduction in the amount of hydrochloric acid in the gastric juice with a consequent reduction of the amount of iron absorbed by the small intestine.

See also Dumping syndrome

Postmyocardial infarction syndrome

Other name Dressler syndrome

Postmyocardial infarction syndrome is a pleuropericarditis occurring 2–12 weeks after a myocardial infarction. Usual symptoms are a sharp severe pain made worse by lying down flat or deep breathing, fever, tachycardia and signs of pleural and pericardial effusions. It is thought to be an autoimmune phenomenon and usually self-limiting.

Postphlebetic syndrome. See Calf pump failure syndrome

Post-trauma syndrome. See Postconcussional syndrome

Post-trauma stress syndrome

Post-trauma stress syndrome is a response to a life-threatening or very dangerous situation, such as a battle, a large disaster, or a physical or sexual assault. Features are likely to be re-living the experience in flashbacks to it or nightmares, attacks of sweating, palpitations, rapid respiration and nausea, by distress when exposed to situations similar to the original one or symbolizing it, hyperalertness or increased startle responses, confusion, dissociation from reality, memory deficits and a loss of interest in work and normal activities. Suicidal thoughts or attempts can occur.

Postvagotomy syndrome

After vagotomy for a peptic ulcer the patient may complain of diarrhoea (which is persistent and severe in about 2% of cases), dumping, weight loss and anaemia.

See also Dumping syndrome

Postviral fatigue syndrome. See Chronic fatigue syndrome

Potter syndrome

Potter syndrome is associated with a failure of fetal urinary production and oligohydramnios (deficiency of the amount of amniotic fluid), which is the cause of a failure of lung development and of limb compression in the foetus. Clinical features are bilateral renal agenesis, pulmonary hypoplasia, skeletal abnormalities, gastrointestinal malformations, and a typical 'Potter facies'.

Pouchitis syndrome

Pouchitis syndrome is inflammation of an ileal pouch, due to an overgrowth of anaerobic bacteria, following colectomy for ulcerative colitis. It occurs in 15–20% of patients.

Prader–Willi syndrome

Prader–Willi syndrome is a relatively common congenital disorder with an incidence of about 1 in 10 000 live births. A deletion from the long arm of chromosome 15 occurs in about 50% of cases and is detectable by gene mapping and by the use of restriction fragment length polymorphs. It is characterized by weak intrauterine movements, breech presentation, hypotonia, delayed attainment of developmental milestones, small hands and feet, small genitalia or undescended testes, overeating and stealing of food, obesity, body-temperature variations, mental retardation, insensitivity to pain, almond-shaped eyes and sometimes cardiovascular abnormalities. Obstructive sleep apnoea due to hypertrophy of the tonsils can occur.

Pregnancy hypotensive syndrome

Pregnancy hypotensive syndrome is an attack of dizziness and sometimes unconsciousness in a pregnant woman in the third trimester of pregnancy when she lies supine and the weight of the foetus compresses the abdominal aorta and inferior vena cava. It is relieved by the woman turning or being turned on her side.

Premenstrual syndrome

Premenstrual syndrome is a complexity of symptoms occurring during the premenstrual period and subsiding with the onset of menstruation. It is not known if it is a disease entity or a form of cyclical phenomena with several different aetiologies. About 95% of women experience some premenstrual symptoms and 20–40% have symptoms severe enough to interfere with their normal activities. The symptoms can include irritability, tenseness, depression, clumsiness, inability to concentrate, weight gain, fluid retention, backache, abdominal bloating, painful and tender breasts, cramps, fatigue, food cravings, appetite changes, frequent micturition and various aches and pains.

Prestomal ileitis syndrome

Prestomal ileitis syndrome is characterized by symptoms and signs of ileal obstruction associated with tachycardia, fever and anaemia. It occurs as a complication of ileostomy for Crohn's disease. There is prestomal contracture of the ileum, with punched-out ulcers, which sometimes penetrate to the serosa.

Presumed ocular histoplasmosis syndrome

Presumed ocular histoplasmosis syndrome is a disease of the eye characterized by peripapillary atrophy of the pigment epithelium, choroidal atrophy and disciform macular lesions. It usually presents in the fourth to fifth decades of life. Neovascularization of the macula follows and atrophic areas develop in the pigmented epithelium. In about a quarter of the cases disciform degeneration affects the fundus of the other eye.

The condition was first recognized in the United States, especially in the Mississippi valley and was attributed to *Histoplasma capsulatum*, a fungus that occurs in the United States but not elsewhere – hence the use of the word 'presumed' for cases arising outside the United States.

Primary antiphospholipid syndrome

Primary antiphospholipid syndrome is related to systemic lupus erythematosus but does not show the full clinical manifestations of that disorder. Clinical features can include arthralgia, migraine, deep-vein thrombosis, pulmonary thromboembolism, arterial occlusions, multi-infarct dementia and livedo reticularis. Antiphospholipid antibodies are present.

See also Sheddon syndrome

Prolapsed mitral valve syndrome

Other name Barlow syndrome

Prolapsed mitral valve syndrome is a form of congenital heart disease in which one or both leaflets of the mitral valve protrude into the left atrium during the systolic phase of ventricular contraction. It is probably the commonest form of congenital heart disease, as echocardiography has shown that it is present in 10–15% of the general population. It can be familial and there is a female:male ratio of 2:1. The mitral valve is affected with a myxomatous degeneration of unknown causation. Clinical features include chest pain, usually sharp and limited to the left side of the chest (which makes it liable to be thought to be angina pectoris due to coronary insufficiency), cardiac arrhythmias of various kinds, and sometimes complete atrio-ventricular block. The characteristic physical findings are a high-pitched systolic click and a late systolic or pansystolic murmur. The average lifespan can be unaffected, but is it reduced by severe mitral regurgitation, severe cardiac arrhythmia or bacterial endocarditis. Sudden death is rare.

Pronator syndrome

Pronator syndrome is a median nerve palsy of the hand due to entrapment of the median nerve between the heads of pronator teres muscle.

Proteus syndrome

Proteus syndrome is a congenital syndrome characterized by thickening of the skin and subcutaneous tissues, subcutaneous masses, vascular disorders, epidermal naevi, and macrodactyly. Other features can be unilateral gigantism, bony prominences of the skull, scoliosis or kyphosis, muscle atrophy, and convulsions.

Prune belly syndrome

Other name Eagle–Barrett syndrome

In prune belly syndrome there is a congenital absence of the muscles of the anterior abdominal wall, and the lax excessive skin of the abdomen looks like the wrinkled skin of a prune. Associated conditions are an enlarged bladder, enlarged ureters, undescended testes, pulmonary hypoplasia and lower limb arthrogryposis (flexion contractures), the last probably due to oligohydramnios. The male:female ratio is 2:1. It can occur sporadically, as an X-linked transmission, associated with chromosomal abnormalities, and as a familial occurrence and is then associated with congenital deafness and mental retardation. Affected girls show only absence of the abdominal muscles. About 20% are stillborn or die within the first 4 weeks of life; 50% die within 2 years. Diagnosis can be made *in utero* by ultrasound by 21 weeks gestation.

Pseudo–Barrter syndrome

Biochemical abnormalities similar to those found in Barrter syndrome can be produced by diuretic abuse or surreptitious vomiting.

Pseudo-bulbar syndrome

Pseudo-bulbar syndrome is one of the 'lacunar syndromes' in which the mutism-anarthria syndrome is associated with bilateral spasticity, bilateral Babinski's sign, a short-stepping gait and inappropriate paroxysms of laughter and crying.

Pseudo-exfoliation syndrome

In pseudo-exfoliation syndrome flakes of basement membrane-like substance from the lens of the eye are deposited onto the anterior lens capsule and the margin of the pupil and in the trabecular meshwork of the ciliary body. This causes glaucoma in about 60% of the eyes. Glaucoma can also occur in the otherwise unaffected eye.

Pseudo-obstruction syndrome

Other name Chronic ileus

Pseudo-obstruction syndrome is characterized by atony of the gastrointestinal wall and gaseous dilatation especially of the colon; the stomach and small bowel may be affected. The diaphragm is pushed upwards and the patient is severely breathless. It can be idiopathic, especially in old people; it can be a side-effect of some drugs (tricyclic antidepressants, morphine, diuretics); it can be a complication of metabolic diseases (hypokalaemia, hypochloraemia), of neurological diseases (multiple sclerosis, diabetic neuropathy, tabes dorsalis, dystrophia myotonia), of endocrine diseases (Addison's disease, hyperparathyroidism, myxoedema), and of amyloidosis, Hirschsprung's disease, disseminated lupus erythematosus, scleroderma, dermatomyositis, lead poisoning, and uraemia.

Punch drunk syndrome

Punch drunk syndrome is characterized by tremor of the hands, epileptic fits, dysarthria (imperfect articulation), slow movements, unsteady gait and a progressive dementia. It is due to degenerative lesions of the cerebral hemispheres and is a disease of boxers as the result of frequent blows to the head and falls on the ring and of jockeys who have fallen frequently. Impaired vision due to cataracts can be a complication.

R

Rabbit syndrome

Rabbit syndrome is characterized by rapid regular involuntary orofacial movements (like the twitching of a rabbit's nose) which are produced by a prolonged use of neuroleptics. The tongue and the rest of the body are not involved.

Radicular syndrome

Radicular syndrome is a unilateral paresis of the abdominal wall with pain, paraesthesiae, hyperaesthesiae and loss of reflexes, due to pressure on a nerve root by a herniation of a spinal disc.

Ramsay Hunt syndromes

There are two variants.

1. *Other name* Geniculate herpes

   Herpes zoster of the ganglion of the facial (seventh cranial) nerve causes pain in the ear, vesicles in the external auditory meatus and fauces and loss of taste. Facial paralysis and vertigo can occur.

2. *Other name* Dyssynergia cerebellaris myoclonica

   This syndrome is characterized by cerebellar ataxia, myoclonus, and occasionally epileptic fits. The cause is uncertain; it may be due to a degeneration of the olivodentatorubral system. It has been classified under the spinocerebellar degenerations and referred to as a form of progressive myoclonic epilepsy.

Rape trauma syndrome

Rape trauma syndrome is characterized by immediate and long-term features. Immediate features are likely to be extreme fear (which may paralyse resistance), feelings of helplessness, or loss of personal integrity and dignity, of being defiled and fear of infection (especially AIDS) and pregnancy. The woman may be left distraught and unable to give a clear and accurate account of what happened. Her feelings may be hidden behind an appearance of frozen calm as if she were distancing herself from the attack. Later features are likely to be fear of going out alone, fear of strangers, flashbacks, nightmares, mood swings, crying fits, loss of appetite and sleep, an obsessive rumination on the attack, withdrawal from previous interests and work, and a loss of desire for sexual relations or a fear of them. With counselling and advice a substantial degree of recovery should occur within several weeks or months.

See also Post-trauma stress syndrome

Raynaud syndrome

Raynaud syndrome is usually seen in young women and has been attributed to an abnormal reaction of digital blood vessels to cold and to sympathetic overactivity. The hands are usually affected, and in some patients the feet can be involved. Characteristic features are bilateral and symmetrical paroxysms of pallor, coldness and numbness on exposure of the digits to cold. The fingers can go into a prolonged painful spasm. The process is reversed by warming, but during the warming there may be intense flushing of the skin with pain and oedema. Complications can be atrophy of the skin and pulps of the fingers, paronychia and ulceration of the fingers.

Recklinghausen syndrome

Other name Von Recklinghausen syndrome (a common but incorrect version); neurofibromatosis

Recklinghausen syndrome is characterized by (a) multiple neurofibromas on nerve trunks, nerve plexuses, cranial and spinal nerves – sarcomatous changes can develop in them; (b) *café au lait* spots or larger pigmented areas in the skin; (c) sessile or pedunculated polyps and swellings of the skin. An acoustic neurofibroma can cause deafness, facial weakness and anaesthesia in the distribution of the trigeminal nerve on the same side. A neurofibroma within the orbit can cause proptosis and visual failure. An optic nerve glioma is an association; it is slow-growing and most likely to occur in childhood.

Recurrent erosion syndrome

Recurrent erosion syndrome is characterized by sudden attacks of sharp pain in the eye, with recurrence in a previously affected area. There is usually a history of corneal abrasion caused by a fingernail, a twig or a piece of paper.

Red diaper syndrome

Soiled children's diapers left unwashed for over 24 hours can turn red due to the red pigmentation produced by *Serratia marcescens*.

Red man syndrome

Red man syndrome is an intense erythema and hypotension produced by rapidly administered vancomycin or amphotericin B.

Refetoff syndrome

Refetoff syndrome is a form of familial thyroid hormone resistance with hypothyroidism or euthyroidism (normal thyroid function), raised thyroid hormone levels, and deaf–mutism.

Refsum syndrome

Other name Heredopathia actictica polyneuritiformis

Refsum syndrome is an autosomal recessive inherited disorder beginning in childhood or adolescence. There is a deficiency of the enzyme phytanic acid α-hydroxylactase, a high blood phytanic acid level, and excessive amounts of phytanic acid in the brain, nerves, heart, liver and kidney. Clinical features include hypertrophic neuropathy, retinitis pigmentosa, cerebellar ataxia, sensorineural deafness, cataracts, icthyosis of the skin, cardiac myopathy, and abnormalities in the electrocardiogram. Death is likely in early adult life.

Reifenstein syndrome

Reifenstein syndrome is similar to Klinefelter syndrome but the XY chromosome pattern is normal. Clinical features are gynaecomastia and a mild degree of feminization. The testes and androgen levels are near normal.

Reiter syndrome

Other names Reactive arthritis; sexually-acquired reactive arthritis; postdysentery arthritis

Reiter syndrome is an association of arthritis, conjunctivitis and urethritis and cervicitis. It can occur after infection by *Shigella flexner, Salmonella typhimurium, Yersinia enterocolitica, Campylobacter jejuni, Chlamydia trachomatis*. Class I antigen HLA-B27 is present in 60–80% of patients (it occurs normally in less that 10% of the population). It can be associated with AIDS. It can follow a non-gonococcal urogenital infection usually due to *Chlamydia trachomatis* or an attack of dysentery. The sexually-transmitted form is most common in young sexually-active men. The postdysenteric form occurs most commonly in women and can occur in children. Clinical features are several.

1. Arthritis. This occurs 3–6 weeks after infection. It usually occurs in the knees, ankles and interphalangeal joints. It can be associated with enthesitis at the base of the calcaneus or at the insertion of the Achilles tendon into the calcaneus, with tendonitis of the Achilles tendon, planter fasciitis and dactylitis of the fingers.

2. Urethritis. This occurs 1–15 days after sexual intercourse. Men can develop balanitis, prostatitis and cystitis, which can be haemorrhagic.

3. Cervicitis in women.

4. Conjunctivitis in one or both eyes. Occasionally keratitis, corneal ulceration, scleritis, uveitis or iritis can develop. About 3% of patients have permanently-reduced vision or blindness.

5. Stomatitis.

6. Keratoderma blenorrhagica. Hyperkeratosis of the soles of the feet and sometimes of the palms, with macules, papules and pustules.

7. Thickened nails with pus forming beneath them.

8. Cardiac disease. Conduction lesions, heart block, murmurs, aortic incompetence, pericarditis.

9. Cranial nerve lesions and peripheral neuropathy.

10. In some patients the illness can present with fever, rigors, tachycardia and very tender joints.

The illness can be self-limiting; it can have multiple recurrences; it can follow a continuous course. Repeated attacks over several years are common, and about 40% of patients are left with a chronic and disabling arthritis, heart disease or impairment of vision.

Remnant particle syndrome

Other names Remnant hyperlipidaemia; dysbeta lipoproteinaemia

Remnant particle syndrome is due to a genetic defect of apolipoprotein E3. There is a rise in cholesterol and triglyceride plasma levels due to an accumulation of cholesterol-rich very low density lipoprotein (VLDL). The increase in cholesterol is due to an accumulation of remnant particles from the hydrolysis of chylomicrons and VLDL, particles which are normally removed by the liver but cannot in this condition be removed owing to the genetic defect. Clinical features can occur in childhood. Planar xanthomas (yellow or orange coloured streaks in the palmar creases) and tuberous xanthomas (short tissue xanthomas) on the elbows and knees are characteristic features. Coronary heart disease, peripheral vascular disease and cerebrovascular disease can occur in the 40s and 50s. In young slim people the prognosis may be better and the only sign they may show is a moderate hypertriglyceridaemia. Associated conditions are glucose intolerance, obesity and hyperuricaemia. The syndrome may be precipitated by renal disease, diabetes mellitus and hypothyroidism.

Rendu–Osler–Weber syndrome

Other name Hereditary haemorrhagic telangiectasia

Rendu–Osler–Weber syndrome is a hereditary disorder transmitted as a single dominant, affecting both sexes equally and appearing in adult life. Telangiectases (clumps of dilated blood vessels) appear on the face, lips and conjunctiva and in the mucous membrane of the mouth. They may vary in size from tiny to half a centimetre across. Bleeding from them occurs and epistaxis and haemoptysis are common. Arteriovenous aneurysms can be present in the intestinal tract, lungs and central nervous system. Iron deficiency anaemia can be produced by the blood loss. Haemothorax is a rare complication.

Repetitive strain syndrome

Repetitive strain syndrome is a general term used to describe various musculoskeletal symptoms such as minor aches, pain or dysfunction of the arm following repetitive or forceful movements occupationally associated. Such symptoms may last for months or years.

Residual ovary syndrome

Residual ovary syndrome is abdominal pain due to enlargement of an ovary which has been conserved during hysterectomy. Cystic enlargement of the ovary, perioophoritis, and pelvic adhesions may be present, and malignant changes can occur in 3%.

Respiratory distress syndrome, infant

Other name Hyaline membrane disease

Respiratory distress syndrome is due to an inadequate amount of surfactant in the lungs of a neonate. Surfactant, a mixture of phospholipoproteins, reduces surface tension in the lungs and permits the expansion of the gas-exchange area in them. It is secreted by the foetal lung from the 20th to the 25th weeks of gestation, with a surge of secretion just before birth in a full-term baby. The syndrome is most likely to occur in a premature baby, a baby of a diabetic mother and a second twin. Its severity varies with the degree of maturation of the lungs at birth. The baby may appear normal at birth with good Apgar scores (for skin colour, muscle tone, respiratory effort, heart rate and response to stimulation), but within a few hours develops tachyapnoea (over 60 breaths per minute), expiratory grunting and sternal recession. Severely affected babies can be cyanosed from birth and have little or no respiration.

Steroids, such as betamethasone and dexamethasone, taken by the mother reduce the incidence of respiratory distress syndrome by stimulating respiratory maturity and the synthesis of surfactant. Aminophylline can be given for the same reason.

Restless legs syndrome

Other name Ekbom syndrome

Restless legs syndrome is an unpleasant creeping sensation of the lower legs with a desire to move the legs to relieve it, with twitching and jumping of the legs. The aetiology is unknown; it may be a subclinical neuropathy or myelopathy. It is a common complication of pregnancy. Fatigue, anxiety and stress are associated factors.

Rett syndrome

Rett syndrome is a progressive encephalopathy with mental deterioration occurring in girls between the ages of 6 and 12 months; previous to the onset they had appeared to be normal. Head growth decelerates, growth is retarded and, in time, previously acquired skills are lost, stereotyped hand-washing movements of the hands occur and autistic features may develop. They can have epileptic seizures of various kinds and 'funny turns'. Seizures can be induced by hypocapnia. Hyperventilation in the awake state can occur and induce non-epileptic seizures. Panic attacks can occur. The electroencephalogram (EEG) is likely to show an increased frequency of spikes, particularly at night with increasing age.

Revolving door syndrome

Revolving door syndrome describes the premature discharge of a psychiatric patient from hospital with his rapid readmission, a cycle which may be repeated several times.

Reye syndrome

Other name Fatty liver with encephalopathy

Reye syndrome is an acute and sometimes fatal illness of children up to the age of 15 years. Fatty degeneration of the liver is associated with acute encephalopathy and neurological symptoms and signs similar to those of the hepatic encephalopathy syndrome. Jaundice is usually absent or minimal, although the liver is enlarged. The serum transaminases and lactic dehydrogenase and blood ammonia concentrations are raised, and in very severe cases acid-base disturbances, hypoglycaemia and coagulation abnormalities can occur. The cause is uncertain. There is a link with aspirin, and the incidence is reduced when parents stop giving aspirin to young children for mild febrile illnesses. It has been associated with viral infections, in particular with varicella, influenza A and influenza B and it may then be due to a circulating toxin from the virus or a substance formed in virus-infected cells. There is an association with juvenile arthritis.

Reye-like syndrome

Reye-like syndrome is characterized by acute hepatic failure and features similar to those of Reye syndrome and is produced by sodium valproate.

Richner–Hanhart syndrome

Other name Oregon tyrosinaemia

Richner–Hanhart syndrome is due to a deficiency of hepatic tyrosinase aminotransferase. Tyrosinaemia is associated with corneal dystrophy, short phalanges, mental retardation and keratoses on the knees, palms and soles occurring within the first few months of life.

Rieger syndrome

Rieger syndrome is a genetically determined syndrome, most frequently as a dominant, but sporadic cases are seen and this suggests a recessive pattern also. It is characterized by a posterior embryotoxon (an opaque ring at the margin of the cornea), a prominent Schwalbe's line (the peripheral edge of Descemet's membrane), adhesions of the iris to Schwalbe's line, and glaucoma. Other features can be hypertelorism (wide spacing of the eyes), hypoplasia of the malar bones, congenital absence of some teeth and mental retardation.

Right upper quadrant syndrome

Right upper quadrant syndrome is a complication of sickle cell anaemia.

Clinical features are fever, vomiting and pain in the right upper quadrant of the abdomen, due to cholecystitis, biliary tract obstruction by gallstones, intrahepatic sickling, urinary tract infection, pneumonia or a vaso-occlusive crisis.

Riley–Day syndrome

Other name Familial dysautonomia

Riley–Day syndrome is an autosomal recessive inherited condition of peripheral autonomic dysfunction due to an enzyme defect in the metabolism and function of catecholamines and occurring mainly in Ashkenazi Jewish children. Clinical features are apparent in the 1st year of life. They include: retardation of physical and mental development, diminished or absent lacrimation, corneal ulceration, excess sweating, frequent fever with poor temperature control, febrile convulsions, anoxic seizures, blood pressure instability with hypertension or postural hypotension, impaired sensation, poor muscle co-ordination, faulty speech, bouts of vomiting, scoliosis and respiratory infections. Death in the 1st year of life is common and is often due to aspiration pneumonia.

Ritter syndrome. See Scalded skin syndrome

Robert syndrome

Robert syndrome is an autosomal recessive inherited disorder characterized by tetraphocomelia (absence of the long segments of all the limbs), cleft lip, cleft palate and cataracts.

Rokitansky–Küster–Haüser syndrome. See Mayer–Rokitansky–Küster syndrome

Romano–Ward syndrome

Romano–Ward syndrome is an autosomal dominant condition with a prolonged Q-T interval on an electrocardiogram and a delay of polarization. Paroxysmal ventricular fibrillation or tachycardia, fainting fits and syncope can occur. Sudden death can occur in childhood, and death during the induction of an anaesthetic can occur at any age. Deafness is not a feature.

See also Idiopathic long Q-T syndrome; Jervell–Lange–Nielson syndrome

Romberg syndrome

Romberg syndrome is a facial hemiatrophy, with which may be associated a localized patch of scleroderma in the frontal region of the scalp, causing a patch of cicatricial alopecia (called a 'coup de sabre' because it resembles the scar of a wound made by a sabre).

Rosai–Dorfman syndrome

Other name Sinus histiocytosis with massive lymphadenopathy

Rosai–Dorfman syndrome presents with bilateral massive painless lymphadenopathy in the neck; lymph nodes may be enlarged in other places. Extranodal lymph tissue has been reported in about one third of the patients – in the skin, lungs, bone, orbits, eyelids, kidneys, peritoneum, testes and the central nervous system. The liver and spleen are not usually enlarged. Other features are fever, weight loss, tonsillitis and nasal discharge and obstruction. The aetiology is unknown. It runs a long course with remissions.

Rotator cuff impingement syndrome

Other names Coracoid impingement syndrome; supraspinatus syndrome

Tendonitis and degeneration in the rotator cuff muscles of the shoulder joint cause pain and limitation of movement. The lesser tubercle of the humerus can impinge on the coracoid process of the scapula. It is an overuse disability with an insidious onset, and is likely to occur in baseball pitchers, javelin throwers, swimmers, tennis players and badminton players.

Rothmund–Thomson syndrome

Other names Rothmund syndrome; congenital poikiloderma; poikiloderma atrophicans with cataract

Rothmund–Thomson syndrome is an autosomal recessive condition characterized by poikiloderma (a mottled appearance of the skin due to mixed pigmentary and atrophic changes), telangiectasia (clumps of dilated blood vessels), cataracts appearing in childhood, alopecia, sparse eyebrows and eyelashes, sparse or absent axillary and pubic hair, hypogonadism and, sometimes, congenital bone defects.

Rotor syndrome

In this disorder of bilirubin, hyperbilirubinaemia is due to a defect in the excretion of unconjugated bilirubin into the biliary caniculi with the bilirubin being reabsorbed into the blood and excreted in the urine. The stools are usually of normal colour. It is diagnosed by liver function tests and liver biopsy. As steroid metabolism is blocked and ovarian steroids undergo metabolism in the liver, oral contraceptives can be a risk.

Roussy–Lévy syndrome

Other name Hereditary areflexia ataxia

Roussy–Lévy syndrome is an inherited ataxia with muscle wasting, pes cavus, kyphoscoliosis and absence of tendon reflexes. It begins in childhood and runs a relatively benign course.

Rubella syndrome

Maternal rubella can cause serious foetal defects, especially if the mother is infected during the first 12 weeks of pregnancy. The usual features are low birth weight, congenital heart disease (pulmonary stenosis, patent ductus arteriosus), microcephaly, deafness and eye defects (microphthalmia, cataracts, glaucoma). Other features can be an enlarged liver, jaundice, an enlarged spleen, purpura, thrombocytopenia (reduction in the number of platelets), myocarditis and encephalitis.

A 'late onset' rubella syndrome can occur. The affected infant shows minimal signs at birth, and at the age of 3 to 6 months develops a multisystem disease with diarrhoea, a skin rash, pneumonia and hypogammaglobulinaemia circulating immune complexes. Later complications can be diabetes mellitus, fits and hypotonia. The rubella virus can persist for a long time in the child's body fluids.

Rubella vaccine syndrome

Two syndromes have been reported as occurring 10–70 days after rubella vaccination. In one, the children developed nocturnal pains and paraesthesiae in the hands and wrists. In the other they had pain in the knees. Mixed cases can occur and in both syndromes there may be polyneuropathy. Symptoms last from 1 day to 5 weeks.

Rubinstein–Taybi syndrome

Other name Broad thumb syndrome

Rubinstein–Taybi syndrome is characterized by multiple congenital abnormalities: microcephaly, an abnormal face (with a prominent forehead, a thin beaked nose, anti-mongoloid slant of the eyes), high arched palate, low-set ears, cataracts, short stature, cardiac abnormalities, hirsutism, renal abnormalities, broad thumb and big toe, haemangiomas of the skin, a failure to thrive and mental retardation. There may be some chromosomal abnormalities.

Rud syndrome

This name is given to any neurocutaneous condition characterized by icthyosis of the skin, epilepsy, short stature, hypogonadism and severe mental retardation.

Rumination syndrome

In this form of hiatus hernia the stomach contents are regurgitated into the mouth by an infant, chewed and re-swallowed.

Russell–Silver syndrome

Russell–Silver syndrome is an autosomal recessive condition characterized by a small triangular face, short stature, abnormally curved fingers, *café au lait* spots on the skin, webbed toes and mental retardation. Asymmetry of the body can occur, one side being larger than the other, and one leg can be larger than the other. Nephroblastoma can be a complication.

S

Saethre–Chotzen syndrome

Other name Acrocephalosyndactyly type III

Saethre–Chotzen syndrome is a congenital condition characterized by acrocephaly (a high pointed skull), which may be asymmetrical, partial syndactyly of digits 1–2 or 3–4 and failure of descent of one or both testes. Other features can be hypertelorism, strabismus, low-set ears, defect of the lacrimal ducts, highly-arched palate, mild hearing loss and bending of the fingers medially or laterally.

Sandifer syndrome

Sandifer syndrome is an association of hiatal hernia, gastro-oesophageal reflux, torticollis and body posturing (such as shaking, body stiffening, hyperextension of the limbs) followed by limpness or apnoea. The hiatal hernia is not always present. Complications are aspiration pneumonia, haematemesis and oesophageal stricture.

Sanfilippo syndrome

Other name Mucopolysaccharidosis type III

Sanfilippo syndrome is an autosomal recessive disease of muco-polysaccharide metabolism characterized by coarse features, joint stiffness and severe mental retardation. It can be due to a deficiency of heparan-N-sulphatase (type A), of N-acetyl-α-D-glucosaminidase (type B), of α-glucosaminidase (type C) or of N-acetyl-α-glucosaminide-6-sulphatase (type D). The biochemical forms are not clinically distinguished.

Savant syndrome

Savant syndrome is an association of severe mental retardation (IQ below 30) with a phenomenal memory for certain events, dates, and the like, and often with an ability to perform very well, often above average ability, in certain limited subjects such as mental arithmetic, calendar calculations and music. The ability to perform in this way usually begins between 5 and 8 years of age and can appear suddenly and disappear without obvious reason. The male–female incidence is about 6:1. The phenomenon has never been adequately explained; possibly it is due to some particular development in the right cerebral hemisphere in an elsewhere badly developed brain.

Scalded skin syndrome

Other names Staphylococcal skin syndrome; Ritter syndrome

Scalded skin syndrome is due to an epidermolytic toxin of certain phage types of *Staphylococcus aureus*. It is mainly a disease of neonates and young children, especially in the first 3 months of life, and is a complication of a staphylococcal infection, usually of the nose, ear or conjunctiva. It can occur in two forms.

1. A generalized form (Ritter syndrome) with a rash, cutaneous tenderness and then the appearance of many bullae. When the epidermis is shed, the child looks as if he/she has been scalded. Temperature regulation and fluid balance are problems.

2. A localized form (bullous impetigo) without cutaneous tenderness and with localized bullae on the exposed parts of the body and around body orifices. This form can progress to the generalized form.

In both forms the bullae normally heal within 7–10 days. Involvement of mucosae is rare. Spontaneous recovery is usual, but sepsis, cellulitis and pneumonia can be complications, and there is a mortality rate of 2–3%.

Scalded skin syndrome is rare in adults, occurring almost exclusively in patients with renal failure who develop a staphylococcal infection, with a build-up of the toxin.

Scalenus syndrome

Other names Scalenus anticus syndrome; Naffziger syndrome

Compression of the subclavian artery or the lower cord of the brachial plexus between a cervical rib and the scalenus anticus muscle can cause pain in the shoulder, extending down the arm, together with wasting of the small muscles of the hand.

Scheie syndrome

Other name Mucopolysaccharidosis type I

Scheie syndrome is an autosomal recessive inherited disease of mucopolysaccharide metabolism in which there is a deficiency of α-L-iduronidase. Clinical features include short stature, coarse features, cataracts, enlarged liver and spleen, stiff joints and, later in life, aortic incompetence. Sleep apnoea can occur. Life span and intelligence are normal. Patients with this syndrome are not as severely affected as those with Hurler syndrome.

Schinzel–Giedion syndrome

Schinzel–Giedion syndrome is a probably autosomal recessive disorder characterized by severe mid-face retraction, bulging forehead, multiple skull anomalies, club-feet, and cardiac and renal malformations. Other features can be excessive growth of hair, six fingers or toes on one limb, phalangeal dysplasia, hypoplasia of dermal ridges, skeletal anomalies in the skull, hands and feet (visible on X-ray), convulsions, growth retardation, failure to thrive, and death in infancy or early childhood.

Schmidt syndrome I

Other name Polyglandular deficiency

Schmidt syndrome was originally described as a combination of Addison's disease and lymphocytic thyroiditis in the same patient. It is now used to describe any combined failure of endocrine glands, including lymphocytic thyroiditis, hypoparathyroidism, adrenal insufficiency, gonadal failure, and diabetes mellitus. An important laboratory feature is the presence of antibodies to one or more endocrine glands.

Schmidt syndrome II

Other name Vago-accessory syndrome

This Schmidt syndrome is characterized by paresis and atrophy of the sternomastoid muscle and part of the trapezius muscle with paralysis of the soft palate, larynx and pharynx on the same side. It is due to a lesion of the nucleus ambiguus in the reticular system and of the nucleus of the spinal accessory (eleventh cranial) nerve. The commoner causes are an infarction or a tumour.

Schüller–Christian syndrome. See Letterer–Siwe syndrome

Schwachman syndrome

Schwachman syndrome is an autosomal recessive inherited disorder characterized by pancreatic insufficiency, reduced neutrophil chemotaxis, and metaphysical dyschondroplasia. Clinical features include short stature, narrowing of the rib cage due to involvement of the ribs, musculoskeletal anomalies, recurrent infections, anaemia, neutropenia and thrombocytopenia.

Schwartz–Jampel syndrome

Other name Myotonic chondrodystrophy

Schwartz–Jampel syndrome is an autosomal recessive myotonic dystrophy disorder characterized by short stature, skeletal abnormalities and an abnormal persistence of muscular contractions.

Scimitar syndrome

An anomalous distended pulmonary vein can present on an X-ray an appearance similar to that of the curved blade of a scimitar.

Seat-belt syndrome

Seat-belt syndrome is any injury of abdominal organs induced by a seat belt in a severe car crash.

Seckel syndrome

Other name Bird-headed dwarfism

Seckel syndrome is an autosomal recessive condition characterized by short stature, a characteristic face (microcephaly, large nose, large ears), joint defects, trident hands, absence of some teeth, a reduction in the number of blood cells and mental retardation.

Sensenbrenner syndrome

Sensenbrenner syndrome is characterized by multiple congenital deformities including short stature, doliocephaly (long head), frontal bossing, hypertelorism (wide spacing of the eyes), short fine hairs, small grey widely-spaced teeth and eversion of the lower lip.

Sertoli cell only syndrome

Other names Del Castillo syndrome; germinal cell aplasia

Sertoli cell only syndrome is a form of hypergonadotrophic hypogonadism in male patients who are infertile but of normal appearance. Germinal cells are absent from the germinal epithelium, but Sertoli and Leydig cells are present.

Sever syndrome

Other name Calcaneal apophysitis

Sever syndrome is a traction apophysitis of the calcaneus at the insertion of the Achilles tendon, provoked by athletic activities and occurring mainly in boys aged 7–10 years. There is pain, tenderness and swelling over the insertion, and the patient limps. X-ray shows fragmentation and increased density of the posterior apophysis.

Sézary syndrome

Sézary syndrome is characterized by erythroderma (abnormal redness of the skin), leukaemia (of abnormally large mononuclear cells), and enlarged lymph nodes (containing the same abnormal mononuclear cells) associated with pruritus, alopecia, oedema and dystrophic nails.

Shaken baby syndrome

Shaken baby syndrome is the result of violently shaking a baby (one form of child abuse). There may be no external signs of injury, but the intracranial injuries include cerebral contusion, cerebral oedema, subdural haemorrhage and subarachnoid haemorrhage.

Sheddon syndrome

Livedo reticularis is complicated by a syndrome of purpura, leg ulcers, scarring, gangrene of toes and transient ischaemic attacks.

See also Primary antiphospholipid syndrome

Sheehan syndrome

Other name Postpartum necrosis of the pituitary gland

Sheehan syndrome is hypopituitarism due to postpartum (occasionally antepartum) necrosis of the pituitary gland due to infarction of the anterior lobe following a severe postpartum (or antepartum) haemorrhage and shock.

Shone syndrome

Other name Parachute mitral valve syndrome

Shone syndrome consists of: (a) a parachute deformity of the mitral valve due to an insertion of all the chordae tendinae into a single pupillary muscle, with blood flow from the left atrium passing through the interchordal spaces, causing various degrees of functional mitral stenosis; (b) a supravalvular mitral ring, an accumulation of connective tissue arising from the atrial surface of the mitral valve with a reduction in the size of the mitral orifice; (c) valvular or subvalvular aortic stenosis; (d) coarctation of the aorta. Heart failure and pulmonary infections are complications.

Short bowel syndrome

Short bowel syndrome is characterized by malabsorption and deficiencies of protein, minerals and vitamins following the resection of a considerable length of small intestine.

Short syndrome. See Sick sinus syndrome

Shoulder-hand syndrome

Other names Reflex sympathetic dystrophy; Sudeck's atrophy; Sudeck–Leriche syndrome

In shoulder-hand syndrome a painful stiff shoulder due to adhesive capsulitis and periarthritis is associated with a diffuse tender swelling of the fingers of the hand of the same side and later with vasomotor changes which causes atrophy of the skin and muscles of the hand. It occurs mainly in old age and can then be associated with other degenerative disorders. The patient can be left with a clawed ankylosed hand and frozen shoulder.

A similar condition can occur as a side-effect of the barbiturates, ioniazid and ethionamide. Burning pain, oedema and decreased sweating of the arm can be followed by contractures of the fingers and dystrophic changes in the nails.

Shulman syndrome

Other name Eosinophilic fasciitis

Shulman syndrome occurs mainly in middle-aged men. The typical feature is a rapid swelling of tender erythematous arms and legs, and later induration of the skin. Other features can be arthralgia, myositis, digital paraesthesiae and Raynaud syndrome. Laboratory findings are eosinophilia, hypergammaglobulinaemia and a raised erythrocyte rate. Spontaneous remissions can occur.

Shwachman–Diamond syndrome

Shwachman–Diamond syndrome is an autosomal recessive inherited disorder in which pancreatic insufficiency (due to fatty degeneration of the gland) is associated with chronic or cyclical neutropenia. Clinical features are malabsorption (due to the pancreatic insufficiency), fever, stomatitis and a risk of severe infections (due to the neutropenia).

Shy–Drager syndrome

Other name Multiple system atrophy with autonomic failure

Shy–Drager syndrome is a disorder of the autonomic nervous system and is characterized by pyramidal disorder, parkinsonism, cerebellar ataxia, bladder and bowel dysfunction, tremor and disturbances of sweating. Respiratory stridor due to paralysis of the abductors of the vocal cords can be a feature. Autonomic neurones are degenerated and there may be atrophic areas in the basal ganglia, midbrain and brainstem. The cause is unknown.

Sicard syndrome

Other name Collet–Sicard syndrome

Siccard syndrome is characterized by paralysis of the palatal, intrinsic laryngeal, pharyngeal, glossal, sternomastoid and trapezius muscles, due to a lesion of the ninth, tenth, eleventh and twelfth cranial nerves.

Sicca syndrome. See Sjögren syndrome

Sick building syndrome

Sick building syndrome is a vague condition with symptoms including lethargy, snuffles, cough, sore throat, headache, itching eyes and influenza-like symptoms. It occurs in office workers in modern buildings. It has been attributed to bad open-plan office design, lack of good ventilation, too many people working in rooms in which the windows cannot be opened, allergy to the droppings of house-dust mites, moulds in air ducts, rays emanating from computer screens, and radon gas seeping through the walls. Legionnaire's disease has been found to be the cause of some cases originally diagnosed as sick building syndrome.

Sick cell syndrome

Sick cell syndrome is characterized by metabolic acidosis, overbreathing, mental disorientation and a low serum sodium. It can be a complication of severe burns, and is thought to be due to a change in cellular membrane properties.

Sick sinus syndrome

Other names Bradycardia-tachycardia syndrome; Short syndrome

Sick sinus syndrome is characterized by alternating bradycardia and tachycardia with outbursts of ectopic atrial tachyarrhythmias and often atrial fibrillation with prolonged periods of sinus node arrests. It has been attributed to a disordered function of the sinoatrial node or deficiency, congenital or acquired, of tissue within the node. Clinical features include dizzy attack, syncope and seizure. It can occur at any age but is most common in old age. Death can occur from biventricular congestive heart failure or auricular fibrillation. In childhood it can be a cause of dizzy attacks, syncope, convulsions and sudden death: no associated congenital heart lesion may be demonstrable.

Silver–Russell syndrome

Silver–Russell syndrome is characterized by short stature, skeletal asymmetry, small incurved little fingers and an altered pattern of sexual development. *Café au lait* macules are present in nearly half the cases.

Sinear–Usher syndrome

Other names Pemphigus erythematosus; seborrhoeic pemphigus

Sinear–Usher syndrome is an erythematous lupus-like rash of the 'butterfly area' of the face associated with superficial scaling or bullous lesions elsewhere. It can be associated with myasthenia gravis and with thymoma.

Sipple syndrome

Other name Multiple endocrine neoplasia II

Sipple syndrome is the sum of the effects of multiple tumours occurring at the same time or consecutively in various organs. These tumours can be: parathyroid adenoma or C-cell tumour, medullary thyroid carcinoma, thymus C-cell tumour, phaeochromocytoma of the adrenal medulla, ganglioneuroma, neuroma and fibroneuroma.

See also Wermer syndrome.

Sjögren syndrome

Other name Sicca syndrome

Sjögren syndrome is a chronic autoimmune disease in which there is a diffuse or focal lymphoplasmacytic infiltration of exocrine glands, which results in diminished secretion and dryness of mucous membranes. Clinical features can include keratoconjunctivitis (due to inflammation and degeneration of the lacrimal glands), a dry mouth (due to a deficient secretion of saliva), dry skin, decreased sweating, dryness and crusting of the nasal passages, blocking of the eustachian tubes which can cause deafness, vaginal dryness which can cause dyspareunia, a patchy alopecia, decrease of scalp and body hair, areas of hyperpigmentation and hypopigmentation of the skin, vasculitis, purpura, cataracts, and Raynaud syndrome.

Sjögren–Larsson syndrome

Sjögren–Larsson syndrome is an autosomal recessive disorder characterized by congenital icthyosis of the skin, followed a year or two later by spastic weakness of the legs, retinitis pigmentosa, dysplasia of dental enamel, and sometimes epilepsy.

Slit ventricle syndrome

Slit ventricle syndrome is characterized by intermittent attacks of headache, lethargy and vomiting in a child with hydrocephalus which is being treated with a shunt. It has been attributed to sudden rises of intraventricular pressure or to the intraventricular catheter being temporarily blocked by pressure against the ventricular wall, the lateral ventricles being so small that they are barely visible on a CT scan.

Sly syndrome

Other name Mucopolysaccharidosis type VII

Sly syndrome is a form of mucopolysaccharidosis characterized by coarse facies, corneal opacities, enlarged liver and spleen, umbilical hernia, inguinal hernia, aortic valve disease, pectus carinatum and joint deformities.

Small-delay syndrome

Other name Simple delayed puberty

Small-delay syndrome is characterized by delayed puberty and short stature, usually in boys, and beginning at 5–10 years as a form of hypogonadotrophic hypogonadism. Later development is normal.

Small left colon syndrome

Small left colon syndrome is characterized by poor development of the descending and sigmoid colon. Obstruction of the bowel can be a complication. The mother of an affected child can be a diabetic.

Small stomach syndrome

Small stomach syndrome is an inability to tolerate large meals after partial gastrectomy owing to the small size of the stomach.

Smith–Lemli–Opitz syndrome

Smith–Lemli–Opitz syndrome is a syndrome of multiple abnormalities: microcephaly, a characteristic facies with micrognathia and anteverted nostrils, short stature, hypoplasia of the thymus, male genital abnormalities, syndactyly and mental retardation. Cardiac, renal and vertebral abnormalities may be present. The eyes may show strabismus, cataracts and ptosis.

Sorsby syndrome

In Sorsby syndrome congenital bilateral macular colobomas are associated with dystrophy of the tips of the fingers and toes.

Soto syndrome

Other name Cerebral gigantism

Soto syndrome is characterized by accelerated growth in the first 4–5 years of life, large hands and feet, clumsiness and mental retardation.

Spitzer–Weinstein syndrome

Spitzer–Weinstein syndrome is a form of distal renal tubule acidosis in which a primary defect in the tubular secretion of potassium causes acidosis.

Splenic sequestration syndrome

In splenic sequestration syndrome there is a sudden pooling of blood within the spleen, which becomes enlarged, with acute hypovolaemia (a decrease in the amount of circulating plasma) and shock. It may have been preceded by a minor febrile illness.

Stagnant loop syndrome. See Blind loop syndrome

Staphylococcal skin syndrome. See Scalded skin syndrome

Steakhouse syndrome

Steakhouse syndrome is an oesophageal obstruction due to a slightly narrowed cardia and the bolting of food.

Steal syndrome

When a large artery is partially blocked, one area supplied by it is temporarily ischaemic as a result of blood having been 'stolen' by another area that is more in need of it.

See also Subclavian steal syndrome

Steele–Richardson–Olszewski syndrome

Other name Progressive supranuclear palsy

Steele–Richardson–Olszewski syndrome is a progressive degeneration of the basal ganglia, oculomotor nuclei and periaqueductal grey matter, of unknown origin and beginning usually after the age of 50. Typical features are a mask-like face with fixed, staring, unblinking eyes, ophthalmoplegia, (paralysis of the muscles of the eyes), nystagmus, unsteadiness, slow movements, frequent falls, pseudobulbar palsy, brisk tendon reflexes, extensor plantar responses and a mild dementia. The patient eventually becomes bedbound and dies within 5–10 years, usually from a chest infection.

Steinert syndrome

Other name Myotonic dystrophy

Steinert syndrome is an autosomal dominant inherited condition characterized by myotonia, muscle atrophy and weakness, conduction defects and arrhythmias of the heart, ptosis, cataracts, strabismus and hypogonadism. Aspiration pneumonia is a complication.

Stein–Leventhal syndrome. See Polycystic ovarian syndrome

Steroid withdrawal syndrome. See Corticosteroid withdrawal syndrome

Stevens–Johnson syndrome

Other names Dry eye syndrome; erythema multiforme major

Stevens–Johnson syndrome is a severe form of erythema multiforme which has been attributed to some foods, drugs, and viral and bacterial infections. About 50% of cases occur in those under 20 years of age, with the more severe forms of the disorder occurring in boys and young adults. In can be associated with malignant disease and systemic lupus erythematosus. There is a maculopapular rash and lesions of the oral, genital and anal mucosa, and haemorrhagic crusting on the lips, associated with fever, headache and arthralgia. Involvement of the eyes can be a deficiency of tears, dryness of the eye surface, conjunctivitis, conjunctival scarring, anterior uveitis, corneal ulceration, symblepharon (adherence of eyeball to eyelid) and panophthalmitis with loss of vision. Pleural bullae can be present and cause pneumothorax and pleural effusion. Other features can be gastrointestinal haemorrhage and ulceration, atrial fibrillation, myocarditis, pericarditis, renal tubular necrosis, nephritis, renal failure, anaemia and fluid and electrolyte disturbance. Death can be due to septi-caemia, pulmonary infection, respiratory obstruction or epidermal necrolysis.

Stewart syndrome

Stewart syndrome is a congenital neurocutaneous disorder characterized by icthyosis of the skin, severe mental retardation, epilepsy, muscular hypoplasia or atrophy, retinitis pigmentosa and arachnodactyly (long spider-like fingers and toes).

Stickler syndrome

Other name Progressive arthro-ophthalmopathy

Stickler syndrome is an autosomal dominant condition characterized by arthritis, cataracts, retinal detachment and glaucoma. Other features can be tall stature, maxillary hypoplasia, a flat facies, deafness, kyphoscoliosis and cleft palate.

Stiff man syndrome

Other name Moersch–Woltmann syndrome

Stiff man syndrome is characterized by a progressive, and at times fluctuating, spasm and rigidity of muscles, starting in middle age and of unknown causation.

Stokes–Adams syndrome

Other name Adams–Stokes syndrome

Stokes–Adams syndrome is characterized by sudden transient attacks of unconsciousness, with or without a fit, due to a temporary cessation of blood supply to the brain, caused by heart-block or bradycardia (heart rate less than 50 beats per minute). It can be due to an overdose of digitalis or to atrioventricular block due to invasion of the atrioventricular node or interventricular septum by a tumour.

Straight back syndrome

Loss of the normal dorsal curvature of the spinal column can compress the heart between the sternum and spine with the production of precordial murmurs and ejection murmurs. Cardiac function is not impaired.

Stress response syndrome

Other name Hoigne syndrome

Stress response syndrome is an acute, immediate and severe reaction to procaine penicillin given intramuscularly. It occurs before the injection is completed or within a minute. Characteristic features are extreme apprehension or fear of death, a feeling of disintegration, a feeling of changes in body shape and weight, visual and auditory hallucinations, rapid pulse, hypertension, cyanosis and sometimes fits. It can subside rapidly, but some patients are left with psychiatric disturbances (fears of a recurrence, fear of any injection, insomnia, distressing dreams, dizziness, loss of concentration) for several years.

Strong syndrome

Strong syndrome is characterized by a familial right-sided aortic arch, asymmetrical facial abnormalities and mental retardation.

Sturge–Weber syndrome

Sturge–Weber syndrome is characterized by capillary or cavernous haemangiomas within the cutaneous distribution of a branch of the trigeminal nerve on one side, associated with a predominantly venous haemangioma of the leptomeninges and cortical destruction beneath it. Complications are convulsions and hemiparesis.

Subclavian steal syndrome

Subclavian steal syndrome is characterized by transient attacks of cerebral ischaemia when the subclavian artery is partially blocked and exercise of the arms produces a reverse blood flow in the vertebral artery.

See also Steal syndrome

Submersion syndrome

Submersion syndrome is cyanosis, confusion, breathlessness and fever in a person who has been nearly drowned. Cardiac arrest can occur. In cold water hypothermia is likely to have preceded the swallowing of water and then the patient is likely to have an amnesia for the event. Pulmonary complications are due to the inhalation of water.

Sudden infant death syndrome

Other name Cot death

Sudden infant death syndrome is the sudden death of an apparently healthy infant. It is a common cause of death in developed countries in the 1st year of life after the neonatal period. Various theories have been advanced about the cause, but no definite cause has been found for the death of an infant under 12 weeks of age. Overheating the baby by too many bedclothes or too hot a bedroom or putting the baby to sleep in the prone position are possible causes. Over the age of 12 weeks the infant may have had a cough or snuffles and the death may be due to a respiratory virus, such as respiratory synctial virus, influenza or para-influenza virus.

Sultzberger–Garbe syndrome

Sultzberger–Garbe syndrome is characterized by severe paroxysmal pruritus with urticarial or follicular lesions progressing to lichenification and most common in middle-aged men.

Superior vena cava syndrome

Superior vena cava syndrome is characterized by dusky skin of the head and neck with dilated veins of the head and neck, dilated superficial collateral veins, and dyspnoea if pulmonary vessels are involved. It can be caused by obstruction of the superior vena cava by a tumour (most commonly a malignant lymphoma, a bronchogenic carcinoma or a lymphoma) and by histoplasmosis and mediastinitis.

Supersensitivity syndrome. See Neuroleptic malignant syndrome

Supraspinatus syndrome. See Rotator cuff impingement syndrome

Surdocardiac syndrome. See Jervell–Lange–Nielson syndrome

Surviving twin syndrome

If one monozygotic twin should die *in utero*, emboli from the dead twin can enter the organs and tissues of the surviving twin and cause microinfarctions.

Survivor syndrome

Survivor syndrome can occur in survivors of concentration camps and major disasters who suffer anxiety, withdrawal, insomnia and nightmares, and feelings of guilt that one has survived when so many have been killed.

Sweet syndrome

Other name Acute febrile neutrophilic dermatosis

Sweet syndrome is of unknown causation, occurs mainly in middle-aged women, and is characterized by painful inflammatory papules, fever, arthralgia and leukocytosis. Some patients are acutely ill. Recurrence can occur. It is sometimes associated with acute myeloid leukaemia.

Swollen baby syndrome

Swollen baby syndrome is characterized by oedema, abdominal distension and respiratory distress in an infant infected with a *Strongylus* worm.

Swyer–James syndrome. See Macleod syndrome

Syringomyelic syndrome

Other name Central spinal cord lesion

Syringomyelic syndrome can be due to syringomyelia or to an intramedullary ependymoma or glioma. The fibres transmitting pain and temperature sense are involved where they cross in the anterior commissure. Usually there is 'dissociated sensory loss', i.e. loss of pain and temperature sensation with relative preservation of touch sensation. Tendon reflexes are usually lost in the affected segments.

Systemic lupus erythematosus-like syndrome

A condition resembling systemic lupus erythematosus can be produced by prolonged treatment with hydralazine in high doses (over 100 mg daily in men, less in women), penicillin and sulphonamides; the condition disappears when the drug is stopped.

T

Tabetic syndrome

Severe 'lightening' pains and loss of vibration and position senses are due to a lesion involving the dorsal horn of the spinal cord. It can occur in tabes dorsalis, diabetes mellitus and meningeal tumours.

Takayasu syndrome. See Aortic arch syndrome

Tangier syndrome

Other name Familial α-lipoprotein deficiency

Tangier syndrome is an autosomal recessive condition in which there is a deficiency of high density lipoproteins. It is named after an island in Chesapeake Bay, USA, where it was first noticed. Plasma triglycerides are raised and cholesterol esters accumulate in reticulo-endothelial cells. The liver and lymph nodes are enlarged and the enlarged tonsils have a yellowish appearance.

TAR syndrome

TAR syndrome is an autosomal recessive condition in which there is an association of:

    T – thrombocytopenia
    AR – absence of the radius.

Severe thrombocytopenia is present in infancy and usually decreases after 1 year of age. Many patients die in the 1st year of life from an intracranial haemorrhage.

Tarsal tunnel syndrome

Compression of the posterior tibial nerve behind the medial malleolus can cause paraesthesiae and pain in the area of the foot supplied by it.

T-D-O syndrome. See Tricho-dento-osseous syndrome

Temporal lobe syndromes

Lesions of a temporal lobe are usually infarction, a tumour or a degenerative disease such as Pick's disease of the brain. Clinical features vary with the position and extent of the lesion and whether the dominant lobe or the non-dominant lobe is affected.

A lesion of the anterior part of a lobe may be asymptomatic. A deep lesion can cause a contralateral hemianopia by involving the optic radiation.

Damage to either lobe can cause aggressiveness and auditory illusions and hallucinations.

Damage to the dominant lobe can cause homonymous upper quadrantopia (blindness or defective vision in one fourth of the visual field), Wernicke's aphasia (failure to comprehend spoken or written language), amusia (failure to recognize or produce musical sounds), dysnomia (partial nominal aphasia) and amnesic aphasia (inability to remember words).

Damage to a non-dominant lobe can cause homonymous upper quadrantanopia, an inability to judge spatial relationships, and impairment in ability to solve tests of visually-presented non-verbal material.

Damage to both lobes (as in degenerative disease of the brain) can cause Korsakoff syndrome and Kluver–Bucy syndrome.

Temporomandibular joint dysfunction syndrome

Temporomandibular joint dysfunction syndrome is characterized by poor movement in the joint with locking and clicking, and pain. It is usually unilateral. It is most likely to occur in women aged 20–40 years. It may be idiopathic or secondary to malocclusion of the teeth or trauma.

Tender oesophagus syndrome

In tender oesophagus syndrome the patient complains that, when he swallows, food sticks in the upper part of his chest. A barium swallow demonstrates a narrowing of the oesophagus caused by pressure from the aortic arch. Narrowing can also occur at the cardia.

Testicular feminization syndrome

Other names Goldberg–Maxwell syndrome; Lubs syndrome; Morris syndrome

Clinical features of testicular feminization syndrome are female external development (including secondary sex characteristics), absence of internal female genital organs, and the presence of testes in the inguinal canal or within the abdomen. There is an end-organ resistance to androgen stimulation. It is the commonest form of male pseudohermaphroditism.

Thalamic syndrome

Other names Central poststroke pain; Déjerine–Roussy syndrome

Thalamic syndrome is characterized by severe scalding, burning or ice-burn and, less commonly, shooting or stabbing pain on the opposite side of the body following a stroke, associated with anaesthesia or adallodynia (pain provoked by a mild stimulus, such as a gentle touch or clothing, but not by firm pressure). It occurs in about 2% of stroke patients.

Third and fourth pharyngeal pouch syndrome. See Di George syndrome

Thoracic outlet syndrome

Thoracic outlet syndrome is characterized by paraesthesiae in the arm, a cold hand and vasospasm due to pressure on the brachial plexus at the root of the neck.

Thrombocytopenia-absent radius syndrome

Thrombocytopenia-absent radius syndrome is an autosomal recessive disorder characterized by thrombocytopenia with or without eosinophilia, absence or hypoplasia of the radius. Other features can be congenital heart disease and strabismus. Death from intracranial haemorrhage occurs in the 1st year of life in about a third of the patients.

Tibialis anterior syndrome. See Anterior tibial syndrome

Tietze syndrome

Other names Costochondritis; costochondral junction syndrome

Tietze syndrome is a painful non-suppurative swelling at a chondrocostal junction, of unknown cause and resolving without treatment. The costochondral junctions are warm, swollen and tender. It usually affects only one side of the chest, and occurs in young or middle-aged adults. It is said to be more common in women than men.

Tiez syndrome

Tiez syndrome is a familial dominant condition in which albinism is associated with deafness and loss of the eyebrows.

Tolosa–Hunt syndrome

Other names Orbital apicitis; ophthalmoplegia dolorosa

Tolosa–Hunt syndrome is characterized by unilateral sharp aching retro-orbital pain, paralysis of the ocular motor nerves (third, fourth and sixth cranial nerves), proptosis and sensory loss over the forehead. It is due to a granulomatous infiltration or an invasive tumour at the apex of the orbit or in the region of the cavernous sinus.

Tooth and nail syndrome

Tooth and nail syndrome is an autosomal dominant inherited condition characterized by absent or peg-shaped primary teeth, absent secondary teeth, absent or small nails and sparse hair.

TORCH syndrome

TORCH syndrome refers to the association of petechiae and purpura with jaundice, anaemia, thrombocytopenia, cataracts, enlarged liver and spleen in a neonate who is small for the gestational age, a condition that can be due to intrauterine infection by:

    T – toxoplasmosis
    O – other infections
    R – rubella
    C – cytomegalovirus
    H – herpes simplex virus.

Touraine–Solente–Golé syndrome

Touraine–Solente–Golé syndrome is characterized by diffuse osteo-thropathy, large hands and feet, periosteal overgrowth and cutis verticis gyrata (corrugated overgrowth of the scalp).

Toxic shock syndrome

Toxic shock syndrome is an acute febrile illness usually produced by a toxin produced by group 1 staphylococcal phage type of *Staphylococcus aureus*. In 85–95% of cases it occurs in women who are menstruating and using tampons, and *S. aureus* has been found in vaginal cultures and sometimes in the blood. Cases unrelated to menstruation have occurred in women, children and men with a staphylococcal infection of a wound, burn, abscess or sinus or as a complication of a chest infection; it is then due to enterotoxin B produced by group 5 type strains. Clinical features are fever with a temperature of at least 38.9°, hypotension with a systolic pressure below 90 mmHg or a diastolic pressure of 15 mmHg or less, renal failure, dizziness, a macular erythematous rash, desquamation, a strawberry tongue, pharyngeal redness, conjunctival redness, vaginal redness, abdominal pain, vomiting and diarrhoea. Leukocytosis and thrombocytopenia are usually present. Other features can be a toxic encephalopathy, myalgia, rhabdomyolysis (death of striate muscle fibres with myoglobin excreted in the urine), and microscopic haematuria. The mortality is about 3%.

It can also be a fatal illness in previously fit young adults due to a toxin produced by group A streptococci.

Transient lazy leukocyte syndrome. See Lazy leukocyte syndrome

Transparent skin syndrome

Transparent skin syndrome is the extreme stage of solar elastosis. Solar elastosis can present with a yellowing, wrinkling, thickening of the skin or, in a fair-complexioned person, with a mottled yellow pigmentation and degeneration of the skin with numerous telangiectases (dilatation of a small group of blood vessels).

Treacher Collins syndrome

Other name Mandibulofacial dystosis

Treacher Collins syndrome is an autosomal dominant inherited condition characterized mainly by maldevelopment of the facial skeleton. The mandible and malar bones are poorly developed and there are abnormalities of the external and middle ear with hearing loss. The eyelids can be notched and the eyelashes are poorly developed in the medial section of the lower lid. There is an anti-mongoloid slant of the eyes. Other features can be cleft palate, congenital deficiencies of the fingers and toes, radio-ulnar synostosis, congenital heart disease and narrowing of the pharynx. Death from respiratory infection is likely in the 1st month of life, but survivors of infancy can have a normal life span.

Tricho-dento-osseous syndrome

Other name T-D-O syndrome

Tricho-dento-osseous syndrome is an autosomal dominant condition characterized by kinky hair, dolichocephaly (long head), dental abnormalities and sclerotic bones and, sometimes brittle nails and brown circular depressed areas of the skin.

Trichlorinophalangeal syndrome

There are two forms of this.

1. Fine brittle scalp hair, pear-shaped nose, abnormally short phalanges, small jaws and dense medial half of the eyebrows.
2. Sparse scalp hair, bulbous nose, microcephaly, abnormally short phalanges, large protruding ears, low intelligence.

Trisomy 13 syndrome. See Patau syndrome

Trisomy 18 syndrome. See Edward syndrome

Trisomy 21 syndrome. See Down syndrome

Trisomy X syndrome

Other name XXX syndrome

Patients with trisomy X syndrome may have underdeveloped secondary sexual characteristics, amenorrhoea and mental retardation.

Tropical splenomegaly syndrome

Other name Big spleen disease

Tropical splenomegaly syndrome, seen in tropical countries, is characterized by an enlargement, often massive, of the spleen associated with lymphocytic infiltration of the hepatic sinusoids. It may be the result of an abnormal immunological response to repeated malarial infection. Other clinical features are fatigue (often to a severe degree) and left upper quadrant abdominal pain. Attacks of acute haemolysis can occur in pregnant women.

True superior oblique sheath syndrome

True superior oblique sheath syndrome is an impairment of upward and medial gaze due to a congenital shortening of the sheath of the superior oblique muscle of the eye.

Tumour lysis syndrome

Tumour lysis syndrome is characterized by weakness, ileus and cardiac arrhythmias following the treatment of large chemosensitive malignant tumours or leukaemia. Other features are hyperkalaemia, hyperphosphataemia, hyperuricaemia, hypocalcaemia and acute renal failure.

Turcot syndrome

Turcot syndrome is characterized by polyposis of the colon and glioblastoma. The polypi vary in number from hundreds to thousands and in size; occasionally they are found in the stomach and small intestine. In the fourth and fifth decades of life they are liable to become malignant.

Turner syndrome

Other name Gonadal dysgenesis

Turner syndrome is one of the most common of chromosome abnormalities. Frequency at conception is thought to be 1.5%, but most affected foetuses abort spontaneously, and the residual birth frequency is between 1/2500 and 1/3500. Common chromosomal abnormalities are: 45XO sex chromosome karytope (51%); mosaics of 45/46 XX sex chromosome (18%); abnormal X chromosome structure (25%). Clinical features include low birth weight, lymphoedema of hands and feet at birth, low stature, incomplete development of the ovaries, incomplete development of secondary sexual characteristics, primary amenorrhoea, low hair line, webbed or broad neck, hypoplastic nails, impaired hearing, an increased carrying angle of the elbows, short fourth metacarpal and metatarsal bones, pigmented naevi and aortic stenosis. Depression to a psychotic degree can be a complication.

Turner–Kieser syndrome. See Nail-patella syndrome

Type A syndrome

In Type A syndrome there is an extreme resistance to insulin in women. Affected women have androgen excess and menstrual abnormalities, frequently associated with polycystic ovaries.

Ullrich–Feichteiger syndrome

Ullrich–Feichteiger syndrome is an association of polydactyly with genital abnormalities.

Uncombable hair syndrome

Other name Spun glass hair

In uncombable hair syndrome the hairs of the scalp are triangular in cross-section with a longitudinal depression along the shaft. The hair will not lie down however much it is combed and brushed. The onset may be in infancy or not until puberty.

Upper limb cardiovascular syndrome. See Lewis syndrome

Urbach–Wiethe syndrome

Other name Lipoid proteinosis

Urbach–Wiethe syndrome is an autosomal recessive condition, a form of lipoglycoproteinosis, with lipid, carbohydrate and protein deposited in the walls of the blood vessels and extracellularly. Clinical features are hoarseness (due to lipid deposit in the vocal cords), papules, nodules, indurated plaques, epilepsy and mental retardation.

Urethral syndrome

In children this presents as a urethritis associated with acute vulvitis or balanitis. In adults it presents as a urethritis and cystitis and sometimes incontinence, with negative cultures; in some there may be a chlamydial infection or a slight degree of urethral stenosis.

Usher syndrome

Usher syndrome is an autosomal recessive disease characterized by retinitis pigmentosa and sensorineural deafness.

Uveal effusion syndrome

Uveal effusion syndrome is a result of a chronic obstruction of the vortex veins of the retina. There is a peripheral choroidal effusion, with thickening of the sclera and an impairment of the blood flow in the vortex veins and often a retinal detachment. The condition occurs in both sexes, usually in the 50s to 70s. Symptoms are at first slight as the effusion is peripheral, but when the retina is detached there is a loss of visual field. The choroidal and retinal detachments can last for months or years but spontaneous resolution can occur.

Uveoparotid syndrome. See Mikulicz syndrome

V

V syndrome. See A and V syndrome

Vago-accessory syndrome. See Schmidt syndrome II

van Bogaert–Epstein–Scherer syndrome

van Bogaert–Epstein–Scherer syndrome is an inherited form of hyper-cholesterolaemia with xanthoma (yellowish lipoid deposits in the skin) and xanthelasmas (similar deposits in the eyelids) associated with mental deterioration, spastic paralysis and cerebellar ataxia due to the deposit of cholesterol in the cerebellum, brainstem and basal ganglia.

van der Hoeve syndrome

Van der Hoeve syndrome is the occurrence of otosclerotic deafness in brittle bone syndrome (osteogenesis imperfecta).

Vasquez syndrome

Vasquez syndrome is a congenital X-linked disorder characterized by obesity, short stature, hypogonadism and mental retardation.

VATER syndrome

VATER syndrome is a syndrome of multiple congenital abnormalities.

    V – vertebral and ventricular defects
    A – anal atresia
    TE – tracheo-oesophageal fistula
    R – radial and renal defects.

There is also a single umbilical artery.

Verner–Morrison syndrome. See WDHA syndrome

Vernet syndrome. See Jugular foramen syndrome

Vertebro-basilar syndrome

The effects of occlusive disease of the vertebral and basilar arteries vary with anatomical variations and on the integrity of the vessels contributing to it or forming it. Occlusion of one artery may produce no symptoms if the other arteries are patent. Occlusion of several arteries can produce ataxia, vertigo, diplopia, visual field defects, deafness, tinnitus, facial weakness and paraesthesiae of the face or arm.

Vibration syndrome

Other name Dead hand syndrome

Vibration syndrome is characterized by blanching and numbness of the fingers and clumsy finger movements, going on to peripheral nerve damage and, rarely, to necrosis of the finger tips in workmen holding vibratory tools, especially in cold weather.

Villaret syndrome

Villaret syndrome is paralysis of the ninth, tenth, eleventh and twelfth cranial nerves in association with Horner syndrome, and due to damage to the nerves by tumours in the posterior retroperitoneal space (such as parotid gland tumours, carotid body tumours, lymph node tumours, secondary tumours) or by tuberculous adenitis.

Visceromegaly syndrome. See Beckwith–Wiedmann syndrome

Visual agnosia syndrome

With a lesion of the occipital lobes, the patient can see but cannot recognize what he sees.

Vitreous wick syndrome

Vitreous wick syndrome is a persistent cystoid macular oedema of the eye which can occur after cataract extraction has been complicated by vitreous incarceration into the incision. It is thought to be due in some cases to vitreous traction on the posterior retina from vitreous strands in the wound; in others it is thought to be due to a low-grade iritis arising from pupillary distortion. There is a slow but increasing impairment of visual acuity.

Vogt–Koyanagi syndrome

Other name Uveomeningoencephalitis

In Vogt–Koyanagi syndrome bilateral inflammation of the iris, ciliary body and choroid of the eye is associated with relapsing meningoencephalitis, deafness, alopecia and depigmentation of the skin and eye. There is a tendency towards recovery of sight, but it is not always complete. The syndrome usually occurs in young adults and in Japanese and Italian men. It is thought to be of viral origin but this has not been proved. If an exudative choroiditis, causing retinal detachment, is present the condition is called Harada syndrome.

Vohwinkel syndrome

In Vohwinkel syndrome, palmoplantar keratoderma is associated with constricting bands of keratin around the bases of the digits, leading to their strangulation and eventual autoamputation, usually during the second decade of life. 'Starfish'-shaped keratoses appear on the dorsum of the hands and feet, and linear keratoses on the elbows and knees.

Volsma–Gons–deViglder syndrome

Volsma–Gons–deViglder syndrome is an autosomal recessive condition due to a complete absence of thyroidal peroxidase. Babies born with this condition have a total inability to organify iodine and are unable to synthesize thyroid hormones.

Von Recklinghausen syndrome. See Recklinghausen syndrome

Vulnerable child syndrome

Vulnerable child syndrome is the chronic anxiety manifested by the parents of a preterm low birth weight infant after discharge from hospital. They continue to regard their child as particularly delicate and fragile and continually having special needs. Child–parent problems can develop, such as difficulty in separation from the mother and feeding problems, and the child can grow up to be over-dependent, demanding and difficult to control.

Waardenburg syndrome

Other names Waardenburg–Klein syndrome; white forelock syndrome

Waardenburg syndrome is an autosomal irregular dominant inherited condition characterized by unilateral or bilateral sensorineural deafness, a white forelock, white eyebrows, a broad root of the nose, lateral displacement of the inner canthus, eyes of different colours and patches of hypopigmentation of the skin. There can be an association with Hirschsprung's disease.

See also Piebald syndrome

Wallenberg syndrome

Wallenberg syndrome is characterized by infarction of the posterior inferior cerebellar artery (which causes ipsilateral paralysis of palatal and pharyngeal muscles), facial anaesthesia and Horner syndrome, and contralateral loss of temperature sensibility and pain sensibility in the limbs and trunk.

Waltman–Walters syndrome

Waltman–Walters syndrome is characterized by right-sided chest or upper abdominal pain, tachycardia and hypotension due to a leak of bile from the gallbladder bed, with an accumulation of bile subhepatically or subphrenically.

Walton syndrome

Walton syndrome is a severe neonatal hypotonia, disappearing in the first decade of life.

Warfarin embryopathy syndrome

The child of a mother who has taken warfarin in the first 3 months of pregnancy may have slight intrauterine growth retardation, hypoplasia of nasal structures, stippled epiphyses, abnormally short fingers and toes, skeletal anomalies, eye abnormalities or connective tissue disorders.

Waterhouse–Friederichsen syndrome

Intravascular coagulation of the blood occurring in meningococcal or pneumococcal septicaemia causes haemorrhages into the adrenal glands with the production of renal failure, vomiting, diarrhoea, purpura, cyanosis, fits and circulatory collapse.

Watson syndrome

Watson syndrome is characterized by *café au lait* macules, axillary and perineal lentigenes (freckles), pulmonary stenosis and low intelligence. It may be a partial LEOPARD syndrome.

WDHA syndrome

Other name Verner–Morrison syndrome

WD – watery diarrhoea
H – hypokalaemia
A – achlorhydria.

The characteristic feature of WDHA syndrome is a profuse watery diarrhoea, the faeces looking like weak tea and rich in potassium thereby reducing the blood potassium level. Other features are confusion, intestinal ileus, abdominal distension and tetany.

Weber syndrome

Infarction or a tumour of the brainstem produces paralysis of the third cranial nerve on the same side and hemiparesis on the opposite side.

Weil syndrome

Weil syndrome is a severe leptospirosis with jaundice, usually accompanied by azotemia, haemorrhages, anaemia, impaired consciousness, and fever. It is probably due to direct damage to leptospires, but it may be an immune response to leptospiral antigens.

Weil–Marchesani syndrome

Weil–Marchesani syndrome is an autosomal recessive disorder of connective tissue characterized by short stature, short fingers and toes, stiff immobile joints, glaucoma and dislocation of the lens. Cardiac abnormalities can be present.

Wermer syndrome

Other name Multiple endocrine neoplasia

Wermer syndrome is the sum of the effects of multiple tumours in various organs occurring at the same time or consecutively. The tumours can be: pituitary adenoma (causing Cushing's disease); adrenal cortical adenoma (causing Cushing syndrome); parathyroid adenoma or hyperplasia (causing hyperparathyroidism); small bowel tumours (causing carcinoid syndrome); insulinoma (causing hypoglycaemia); gastrinoma (causing an excess of hydrochloric acid secretion in the stomach); and somatostatinoma (causing an excess secretion of somatostatin).

See also Sipple syndrome

Werner syndrome

Other name Pangeria

Werner syndrome is an autosomal recessive disorder characterized by cataracts, retinitis pigmentosa, glaucoma, corneal opacities, premature greying and thinning of the hair of the scalp, axillae and pubic region, atopic changes in the skin of the face, limbs, hands and feet, a birdlike facies and short stature due to an arrest of growth at puberty. Associated conditions are arteriosclerosis, diabetes mellitus, malignant disease and hypogonadism.

Wernicke–Korsakoff syndrome

Wernicke–Korsakoff syndrome is an association of Wernicke's disease (ataxia, bilateral ophthalmoplegia, nystagmus, pupillary abnormalities, ptosis, peripheral neuropathy, tachycardia) with Korsakoff syndrome (gross memory defect and confabulation – relating imaginary experiences to fill the gaps in memory), due to vitamin B_1 (thiamine) deficiency, usually in chronic alcoholics. Without treatment the course is downhill to death within a few weeks.

West syndrome

Other name Infantile spasmic epilepsy

West syndrome is a form of epilepsy which usually begins in the 1st year of life and is due either to severe prenatal or perinatal cerebral damage or to tuberous sclerosis. The typical feature is a spasm, consisting of a sudden flexing of the head on the neck, flexion and abduction of the arms, and bending of the knees. Other forms of epilepsy can occur. Mental retardation is an associated feature. The electroencephalogram (EEG) shows hypsarrhythmia (a gross disturbance with random high-voltage slow waves and spikes spreading to all cortical areas).

White forelock syndrome. See Waardenburg syndrome

Whipple's disease-like syndrome

Whipple's disease-like syndrome is characterized by fever, diarrhoea and loss of weight. The bowel walls are irregularly thickened, there is hypersecretion of intestinal fluid, and the stools contain large numbers of acid-fast bacilli.

Wiedemann–Rautenstrauch syndrome

Wiedemann–Rautenstrauch syndrome is a congenital condition probably inherited as an autosomal recessive. Characteristic features are intrauterine growth retardation, failure to thrive, short stature, a progeria-like appearance (i.e. resembling old age), hypotonia, lipoatrophy, and mental retardation. Death occurs before six years of age.

Williams syndrome

William syndrome is a congenital syndrome occurring sporadically in which a high blood calcium is associated with developmental delay, elfin facies, anteverted nostrils, strabismus, dental abnormalities, small nails, supravalvular aortic stenosis, and short stature.

Wilson–Mikity syndrome

Other name Pulmonary dysmaturity

Wilson–Mikity syndrome is characterized by pulmonary insufficiency, cyanosis and hyperpnoea in low birth weight infants during the 1st month of life. The lungs show multiple cyst-like foci (with a 'soap bubble' appearance due to focal hyperaeration) and interstitial fibrosis. It may be due to unequal postnatal development of the alveoli. Other features are slight enlargement of the heart and enlarged proximal pulmonary arteries. Complete recovery is possible, but severe disease can cause death. Radiographic signs resolve within 12 months in the patients who recover.

Wiskott–Aldrich syndrome

Other names Aldrich syndrome; immunodeficiency with thrombocytopenia and eczema

Wiskott–Aldrich syndrome is an X-linked recessive disorder of male children characterized by thrombocytopenia (reduced number of platelets), deficiency of T cells with reduced T-cell function, deficiency of IgM, purpura, chronic eczema and recurrent bacterial and fungal infections. The platelets are small and deficient in adenosine diphosphate (ADP) as a result of which they do not aggregate normally. Thrombocytopenia can cause a bloody diarrhoea and intracranial haemorrhage. Haematuria, proteinuria, increased blood urea nitrogen and decreased creatinine clearance occur in about 20% of patients. The disease usually presents in infancy with bleeding or recurrent infections due to *Streptococcus pneumoniae* or *Haemophilus influenzae*. The bleeding may be slight. Recurrent infections, especially herpes simplex, are likely later, and later in life there is an increased incidence of malignant disease and of non-Hodgkin's lymphoma. The prognosis is poor, with few patients surviving into their teens. Death is likely to be due to infection, haemorrhage or malignant disease.

Wolfahrt–Kugelberg–Welander syndrome. See Kugelberg–Welander syndrome

Wolf–Hirschorn syndrome

A deletion of the short arm of chromosome 5 can be sporadic or familial. Clinical features can be hydrocephalus, cleft lip and palate, cataracts, strabismus and mental retardation.

193

Wolff–Parkinson–White syndrome

In Wolff–Parkinson–White syndrome impulses carried by the bundle of Kent (an accessory pathway between atria and ventricles) pass relatively rapidly from atria to ventricles, bypassing the normal delay imposed by the auriculoventricular junction. This causes a partial early depolarization of the ventricles, which is followed by completion of ventricular depolarization via the normal conduction system. The ventricular depolarization via the bundle of Kent travels through working myocardial cells with a slow conduction velocity. The early depolarization creates an initial slurring of QRS which is called a delta wave. The condition is associated with episodes of supraventricular tachycardia produced by re-entrant pathways involving the auriculoventricular junction at the accessory pathway. The syndrome is described as Type A or Type B, depending on the direction of the delta wave in the EEG.

The condition presents in childhood and is most common in children with congenital heart disease, especially Ebstein's anomaly. Attacks of paroxysmal tachycardia can occur. There is a risk of sudden death.

Wolfram syndrome. See DIDMOAD syndrome

Wolman syndrome

Wolman syndrome is an autosomal recessive form of lipoidosis with an onset early in infancy. Clinical features are diarrhoea, a failure to thrive, enlargement of the liver, spleen and adrenal glands, punctuate adrenal calcification, osteoporosis, and degeneration of the thymus. Death occurs in infancy.

Woolly hair syndromes

There are a number of such syndromes, which are characterized by coil hair in the scalp of a non-black person. The coil hair is present at birth, increases in childhood, and starts to disappear later in life.

Wyburn–Mason syndrome

Other name Racemose angioma

Racemose angioma of the retina is due to abnormal arteriovenous communications being formed during the development of the retinal vessels.

The angioma can extend backwards to involve the optic nerve and midbrain and the condition is then called the Wyburn–Mason syndrome. The blood vessels are massively dilated and there is arterialization of the walls of the veins due to the big blood flow. A slow increase in the size of the vessels can occur over years, and if the optic nerve head is involved vision is gradually lost.

X

X syndrome

X syndrome is an association of insulin resistance with hypertension, hyperinsulinaemia, obesity and high plasma levels of low-density lipoproteins. It is an important factor in the pathogenesis of atherosclerosis and coronary artery disease.

Xanthine syndrome

Xanthine syndrome is premenstrual breast turgidity and tenderness made worse by drinking tea, coffee or coke.

XTE syndrome

XTE syndrome is an autosomal dominant inherited syndrome, characterized by:

    X – xeroderma (dry skin)
    T – talipes
    E – enamel defect of the teeth.

Associated conditions are absent eyelashes, sparse coarse hair, a decrease in the number of sweat glands, dystrophic nails and sometimes bullae in the skin.

XXX syndrome. See Trisomy X syndrome

XXXY syndrome

Other name Barr–Shaver–Carr syndrome

The patient has 48 chromosomes (XXXY karyotype). XXXY syndrome resembles Klinefelter syndrome: tall slim build, delayed puberty, testes small or undescended, small penis, gynaecomastia (excessive breast development in the male) and mental retardation.

XXY syndrome. See Klinefelter syndrome

XXYY syndrome

XXYY syndrome is a chromosomal disorder (XXYY karyotype) and is characterized by delayed puberty, gynaecomastia (excessive breast development in the male), skeletal and cardiac abnormalities and mental retardation.

Y

Yawning syndrome

Other name Pathological yawning

In the yawning syndrome the patient has attacks of uncontrollable yawning lasting for 10–20 minutes. They occur without warning and can be accompanied by a croaking noise. It can be familial. The cause is unknown.

Yellow nail syndrome

Yellow nail syndrome is characterized by slow-growing, thick, yellow or greenish nails, associated with chronic bronchitis and bronchiectasis and with oedema of the legs due to atresia or varicosity of the lymph vessels.

Youssel syndrome

Other name Vesico-uterine fistula

Youssel syndrome is periodic haematuria due to a fistula between the uterus and the bladder, which can occur as a complication of operations on uterine neoplasms and enables menstrual blood to pass into the bladder.

Yunis–Varon syndrome

Yunis–Varon syndrome is a congenital disorder characterized by defective ossification of the skull, partial or complete absence of the clavicles, smallness of the jaws, bilateral absence of the thumbs and first metacarpal bones, absence of the distal phalanges of fingers and toes, vestigial nails, and generalized skeletal changes.

Z

Zellweger syndrome

Other name Cerebrohepatorenal syndrome

Zellweger syndrome is an inherited (probably autosomal recessive) syndrome characterized by imperfect myelinization of nerve tracts, microgyria, calcific deposits in long bones, craniofacial malformations, hypospadias, glaucoma, cataracts, cysts of the kidney, an enlarged liver, hyperbilirubinaemia, extramedullary haemopoiesis and hypotonia. Death occurs in infancy.

Ziehen–Oppenheim syndrome

Ziehen–Oppenheim syndrome is a familial torsion spasm due to a lesion of the basal ganglia. The torsion spasm begins in one leg and gradually progresses to a severe disability.

Zieve syndrome

Zieve syndrome is characterized by acute haemolysis and jaundice in alcoholics with a fatty liver and severe hyperlipidaemia.

Zinsser–Engman–Cole syndrome

Other name Dyskerotosis congenita

Zinsser–Engman–Cole syndrome is an inherited disorder presenting at 5–10 years of age and characterized by painful, slow–healing, recurrent oral ulcers, oral leukoplakia, pigmentation of the skin and dystrophic nails.

Ziprkowski–Margolis syndrome

Ziprkowski–Margolis syndrome is a congenital syndrome of males, characterized by hypopigmentation of the skin with hyperpigmented macules which give the skin a piebald appearance, irises of different colours, and deaf-mutism.

Zollinger–Ellison syndrome

Zollinger–Ellison syndrome is severe and recurrent peptic ulceration due to an excessive production of gastrin by abnormal G cells in the antrum of the stomach or by the cells of an islet-cell tumour in the pancreas. The gastric, duodenal and jejunal folds are large and thickened and the proximal small intestine is dilated. Gastrinomas can be a complication; 50% of them are malignant and metastases can occur in lymph nodes and the liver.

Zondek syndrome

Zondek syndrome is characterized by postpregnancy irregular uterine bleeding, galactorrhoea and hyperthyroidism, and has been attributed to pituitary overactivity.

Authors' note

Although a large number of syndromes are described in this book, the authors are conscious that more exist and that new syndromes are described every year. They would be grateful, therefore, if any reader noticing a significant omission or a new syndrome would bring it to their notice (via the publishers) so that it can be included in the next edition.